The Medieval Leper

and his northern heirs

PETER RICHARDS

BARNES & NOBLE
BOOKS
NEW YORK

This edition published by Barnes & Noble, Inc.,
by arrangement with Boydell & Brewer Ltd.

1995 Barnes & Noble Books

ISBN 1-56619-774-0

Printed and bound in the United States of America

M 9 8 7 6 5 4 3 2 1

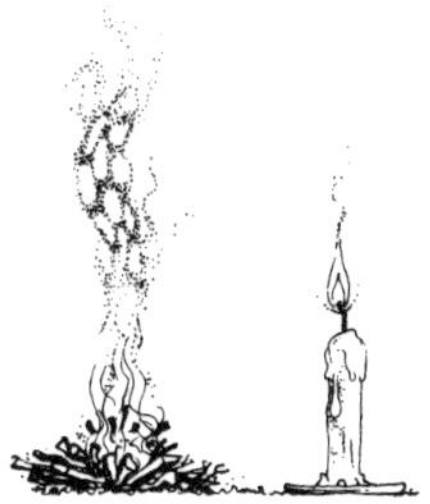

"If any brother or sister leper is so sick that hope is lost, he should have a fire, a candle, and all he needs until he recovers or dies. Then on the day when anyone is buried food and drink should be given to the burial party."

". . . in the house itself they should have four lead cisterns, four pans, four tripods, two tubs, one broom, and a spade for burying the dead."

The Regulations of Sherburn leper
hospital near Durham (founded *c.* 1181)

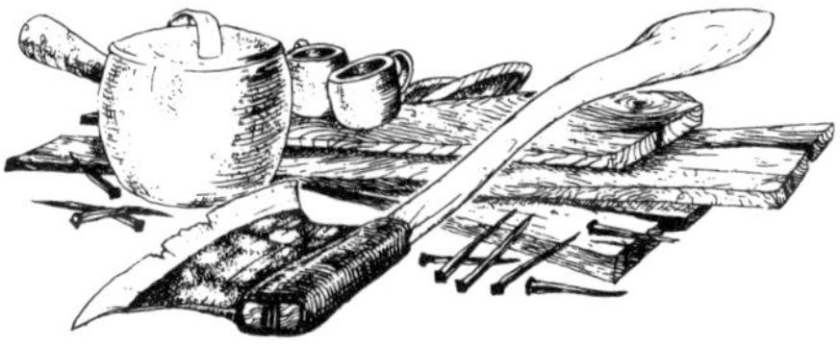

"Maths Bengtson of Fremanby and Erich Hanson of Ökarby are instructed to make ready clothes of all sorts for several years use. Also bedclothes, wood and nails for coffins, axe, cooking pots, drinking and eating utensils . . . so that these sick men can be taken away in the Spring as soon as the crops have been sown."

Report of Pastor Boëtius Muur's visit to the parish of
Saltvik, Åland islands, March 10th, 1658.

"The houses of the lepers in Posta and Bredhbolsta are to be burnt down. A boy in Skarpnötöö who is a leper must be sent to the hospital immediately. The two small leper children in Eckeröö and Stoårby were given 5 D : r from Ekröö and 8 D : r from Jommala almsbox. Two months supply of food was also taken to them from the Jommala Christmas food. Wood and nails for coffins have also been provided for them."

Report of Pastor Boëtius Muur's visit to the parish of
Hammarland, Åland islands, June 21st, 1658.

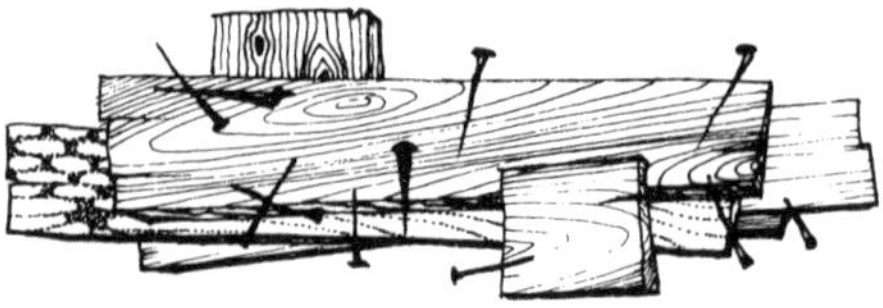

"They say that the old churchyard is so packed full that they could not bury any more corpses there. Because they often lie ill and no more than one or two are up and about, they could not have the graveyard situated far from the houses. It was therefore suggested that the small patch of ground south of the old buildings should be proved with iron rods to see whether the earth is deep enough; when that becomes full up then they must again make use of the old churchyard, if nowhere better is found.

"They need two barrels for cooking oil as soon as possible. . . ."

Report of the inspection visit by
Pastor Boëtius Muur to the leper
hospital at Gloskär, Åland islands,
July 17th, 1665.

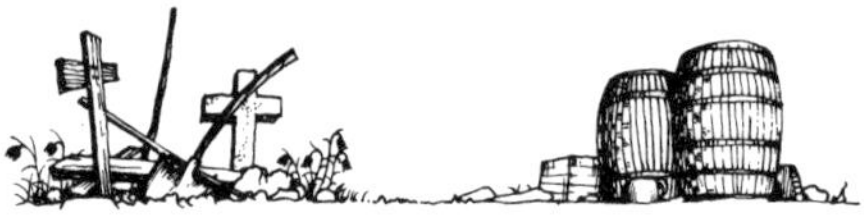

". . . the hospital . . . has manifestly been hitherto a sort of graveyard for the living. . . ."

"With the doctors' best intention, insight and industry it is impossible to heal the living dead. . . ."

". . . the wretched leper . . . must renounce the best of an individual's freedom and rights; happiness flees him as well as life itself, and only death's certain call can comfort and satisfy him."

J. E. Welhaven, chaplain to
St. George's leper hospital,
Bergen, 1816.

Preface

People are the theme of this book—people beneath the notice of history but for their disease: leprosy, or suspicion of it, is their only claim to fame. Medieval history is rich in traditions about what should have happened to lepers, but singularly silent about what actually became of them. A golden opportunity to look into medieval minds through the mirror of medieval suffering has almost been lost.

But something can be saved; the bare bones of history can in fact be given flesh and blood. Both leprosy and its medieval traditions persisted after the Middle Ages in some isolated communities, notably on the Åland islands in the seventeenth century. Here, the personal impact of medieval attitudes to leprosy can be discovered; here, the frightening reality of the individual burden of this disease springs to life.

Both historians and physicians have doubted the medical reality of medieval leprosy. Few people are aware, however, that although the disease disappeared from most of Britain and western Europe in the sixteenth century, it lingered on in an unbroken succession in north-west Europe until a few years ago. This fact, and the bones of medieval Danish lepers, can be used to establish the identity of medieval leprosy beyond reasonable doubt.

No attempt has been made to write a comprehensive account of European leprosy, for in the Middle Ages experience and attitudes were similar throughout Europe. My attention has focussed upon Britain and Scandinavia, countries whose peoples share many traditions and attitudes. Detailed knowledge of Scandinavian geography and history is not necessary, but reference to the maps will help in orientation. The Åland islands between Sweden and Finland, which are central to the story, have been administratively linked with Finland since 1636. Finland was for centuries a province of Sweden, a complicated arrangement of both alliance and subjugation, until, in 1809, Finland was ceded to Russia under a peace treaty, and became an autonomous Grand Duchy of Russia. Finland declared her independence in 1917, an independence she has firmly, wisely, and even fiercely maintained since.

Both Finnish and Swedish are official languages in Finland, but since most of the relevant historical records were in Swedish, the Swedish place-names have been used throughout. Thus Helsinki is referred to as Helsingfors and Turku as Åbo, although these cities are more commonly known by their Finnish names today. The variable spellings of place names have not been altered when original documents are quoted. As for the pronunciation of the many Scandinavian names, the reader is advised to render them as best assists his reading.

The term "leper" is now deprecated both by those who have devoted their lives to the relief of suffering from this disease, and by the World Health Organisation. Their view is justified by the stigma still attached to the name. But this book interprets that stigma: to hide the name by which these unfortunate people were known would not only diminish the significance of events but would, in my view, be an unjustifiable attempt to rewrite history. Yesterday's victims of leprosy were "lepers", with all that the name implies; today's and tomorrow's are "leprosy patients".

Over the years I have received generous help. In my field studies twenty years ago I was particularly indebted to Prof. dr. med. V. Møller-Christensen, the late dr. phil. Svend Larsen, Prof. dr. med. I. Rokstad, Dr. M. Pärmala and Dr. H. Hellberg; the Scandinavian Studies Fund of Cambridge University gave timely financial assistance, and many friends provided generous hospitality. More recently I have been greatly assisted by Dr. L. J. Irgens and also by dr. phil. Knud Larsen. The Swedish Institute in Stockholm and the University of Bergen library kindly provided copies of important source material. Documents in Latin were translated by Dr. B. Dicker and one by Mr. N. R. Hale. The source of photographs are acknowledged in the list of plates, but I am particularly indebted to Mr. Kristofer Gräsbeck, lately Press Counsellor at the Finnish Embassy in London, for help in bringing the Finnish scene to life. I am also most grateful to Dr. S. G. Browne, Director of the Leprosy Study Centre, London, for his opinion on the diagnosis of these historical patients. J. Pfrimmer & Co., Erlangen, gave a generous grant towards the production of the book. Finally, from my wife I have received invaluable secretarial help and assistance with translations of the Scandinavian languages for many years.

In this brief incursion into history I must "confess frankly", as did William Turner in the preface to his *Libellus de re Herbaria* (1538), "that I am unworthy to act as bottle-washer to the most learned.... So my dear reader take this labour of mine with a smile, and if you make any progress by me, nothing will give me more pleasure. If I am caught blundering (and this is very easy) I will gladly be corrected by men of learning. For I am not too proud and pleased with myself to accept gladly the verdicts of the learned. Fare you well."

PETER RICHARDS

Contents

Illustrations

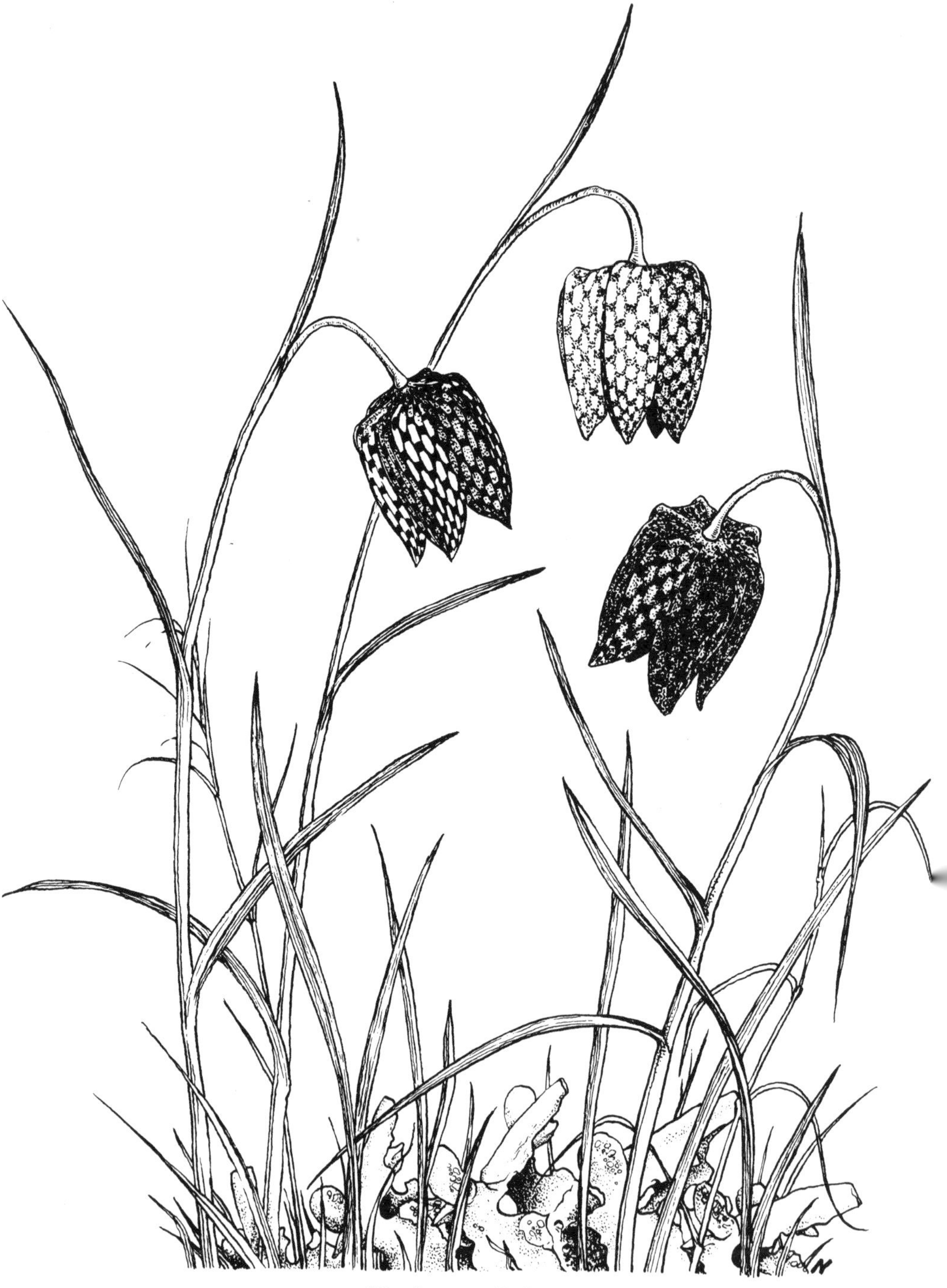

The Lazarus Bell.

INTRODUCTION

Leprosy

Leprosy is unique—both medically and in its place in social history. This book is concerned more with the reality of the impact of a disease upon individuals and communities, than with the medical identity of the disease itself. Unlike the explosive epidemic diseases—plague, smallpox, measles, typhus, and the enteric fevers—leprosy had no national economic or political importance; its burden was personal and local. At the same time, historians should know whether medieval leprosy was as real as those other diseases, for there are several reasons why it might not have been. Neither aspect can be usefully discussed without background knowledge of the disease itself.

No bacterial disease is longer in its gestation, more variable in its expression, or more mutilating in its fullness. Leprosy has many disguises. So variable are its features that it could reasonably be thought to be not one disease but many: its extremes range from a disfiguring skin disease to a mutilating disease of hands and feet. Only with the knowledge that the same bacteria are present in these superficially different disorders can the mosaic confidently be pieced together as one infection. The gross, classical forms of the disease are in fact just the tip of the iceberg of leprosy. But what the twentieth century has only recently appreciated, the Middle Ages cannot be expected to have known. At best, recognition of the most characteristic features of advanced disease is all that can be looked for.

Leprosy is an infectious disease caused by *Mycobacterium leprae*, a first cousin to tuberculosis bacteria. Unlike tuberculosis, leprosy bacteria cannot be grown outside living animal cells, and even within them they multiply very slowly; they can remain dormant, alive but inactive, for a long time. Leprosy bacteria probably spread from person to person as readily as tuberculosis, but disease less often follows, both because the bacteria are less virulent and because most people have a high degree of natural resistance to the disease. Tuberculosis, and probably leprosy too, often causes an infection which smoulders, heals, and is never recognised. When symptomatic leprosy does develop, its incubation period is longer than in any other infectious disease, often being measured in years, not days, weeks or months.

The precise form and progress of leprosy depends partly on the degree of natural resistance to infection, and particularly on both the intensity of the production of antibodies and the reaction of body cells against the bacteria. A strong antibody response often eventually overwhelms the infection, but only at the expense of widespread tissue destruction. Natural resistance does not depend upon antibodies but upon obscure, probably inborn, racial and familial factors: thus the clustering of leprosy in families has a deeper significance than repeated exposure to infection.

The spread of leprosy is still not well understood. Bacteria are shed from infection in the nose, throat, and skin, and these are probably the sites to which they are first transmitted in others. Skin can only be invaded through cuts, scratches, or insect bites, the latter being common in the poverty in which leprosy has thrived. No evidence supports the medieval tradition that leprosy is commonly spread by venereal infection. Nor does that opinion imply confusion between leprosy and syphilis, for which there is no convincing evidence (1). The antiquity of the myth of sexual transmission of leprosy, traced back to ancient China and still current in primitive regions today, is no guarantee of its truth. Most compelling of all the arguments against it is the fact that although leprosy shows a strong family incidence, both husband and wife are affected in less than 5% of couples.

About nine in every ten people infected with leprosy bacteria do not show any signs of disease; some of the remainder have a mild and self-healing infection; a few have more active and extensive disease. If the body reacts strongly to the infection ("high-resistance" leprosy), the skin is not severely disfigured, but nerves are damaged because of an intense reaction around bacteria lodged within them; once fingers and toes become paralysed and feeling is lost, they become easily injured, infected, and mutilated. When, at the other end of the spectrum, there is a singular lack of response to bacterial invasion ("low-resistance" leprosy), the disease progresses unchecked, causing large lumps or patches on the skin, which later disintegrate into discharging sores. The voice becomes hoarse because of infection in the throat. Nerves are destroyed by invasion with large numbers of bacteria, but later than in the high-resistance form of the disease. The eyes are often damaged in both variants, resulting in blindness. Between these two extreme expressions of the disease are many shades of both.

Leprosy was incurable until about thirty years ago. Drugs can now both minimise tissue destruction and eventually cure the disease. Deformities can often be corrected surgically. The key to successful management is early diagnosis and prompt treatment.

THE TRADITION

I

A Cross-roads in History

The Åland islands lie at the northern crossroads of the Baltic Sea. To the West, they guard the approaches to Stockholm; to the East, the Gulf of Finland leads to Helsingfors and, further, to Russia; to the North, the Gulf of Bothnia separates

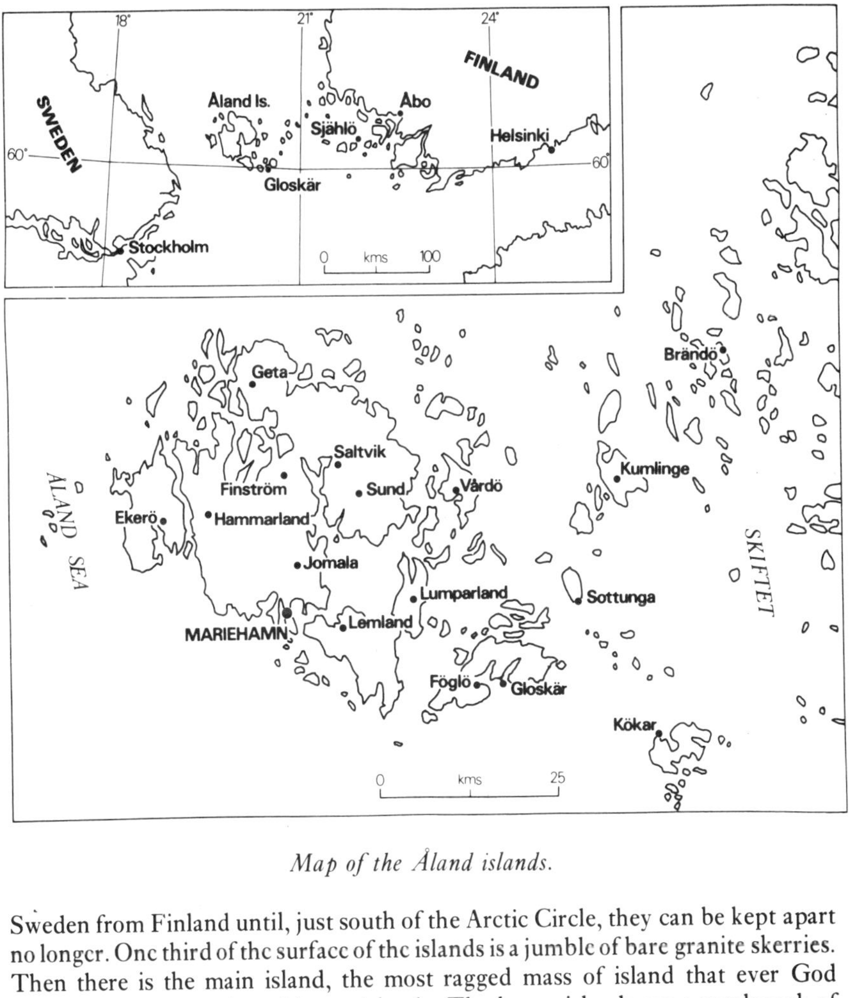

Map of the Åland islands.

Sweden from Finland until, just south of the Arctic Circle, they can be kept apart no longer. One third of the surface of the islands is a jumble of bare granite skerries. Then there is the main island, the most ragged mass of island that ever God created, and a scattering of lesser islands. The larger islands are a patchwork of meadows, boulders and bogs, pine, spruce, and birch. The smaller islands boast only a carpet of moss, cotton-grass, bilberry, crowberry, and heather, with a wind-swept growth of stunted trees and dense juniper bushes. They look today as they have looked for centuries.

These islands not only command the highways of the sea, but they also stand at one curious and forgotten cross-roads in history. Not the history of nations, although they have appeared there, but of individuals: people remembered only because of a catastrophe which destroyed their health, hope, and their very lives—the disease leprosy.

Leprosy was a familiar disease in medieval Europe. As the surroundings and circumstances of the Middle Ages retreated slowly northwards in the sixteenth and seventeenth centuries, leprosy ebbed and eddied with them. The disease not only survived in the slowly changing North, but in the nineteenth century even prospered, continuing in an unbroken succession until very recently.

In many respects the lepers of mid-seventeenth-century Åland lived and died in the Middle Ages. The colour of their church had changed, but little else. By chance, their fate in this medieval microcosm was recorded by Boëtius Muur, dean of Åland, whose diaries (1) were discovered in the archives of the parish of Korpo in south-west Finland in the summer of 1875. Of medieval rules, regulations, and provisions for lepers we know much; of the degree to which they were enforced we know little; of the people themselves we have, hitherto, known next to nothing.

Through Muur's brief jottings the medieval leper can be rediscovered, clothed, and brought to life. From the description of the physical hardships we can imagine something of the leper's despair, but his own thoughts are tantalisingly silent. Not until the early nineteenth century, in another Scandinavian context, are both the full horror in his mind and the depth of his courage authentically revealed; partly through the eyes and ears of Pastor Welhaven of Bergen in Norway, and partly in a poem by Peder Olsen Feidie, a Norwegian leper.

Few historical figures have attracted so much myth and misconception as the medieval leper. For years it was uncritically believed that leprosy was brought to Europe by returning crusaders. But excavations in 1966–73 of a Romano-British burial ground at Poundbury Hill in Dorset uncovered the skeleton of a leper (2). Unfortunately, only the feet and lower legs were found; without other bones, in particular the skull, several rare diseases which may mimic the bone destruction caused by leprosy cannot finally be excluded. The balance of evidence, however, strongly suggests that a leper lived in England in the fourth or fifth century A.D.—a Roman soldier perhaps, or a British camp-follower.

It is entirely credible that leprosy existed in late Roman Britain. Being a slow disease and not very infectious, leprosy might take decades or even centuries to establish itself sufficiently in a community to become the subject of legislation. Yet already in 757, a law was enacted in France concerning the marriage of lepers. Leprosy is mentioned in Irish records from the same period. Later, in 921, the Irish Year Book recorded that when Armagh in Ulster was plundered by the Viking king, Gudrød of Dublin, he spared "the houses of prayer where the men of God and the lepers stayed", an act of mercy which can hardly be attributed to religious scruples. Leprosy is also mentioned in the tenth-century laws of the Welsh king, Hywel Dda. At the same time, a disease was recognised in Anglo-Saxon England which was identified with Latin descriptions of leprosy. Aelfric, archbishop of Canterbury, alluded to "*seó miccle códu* which leeches (doctors) call *elefantinus morbus*" (3). Several other references to this disease, to *seó mycle adl*, and to "the great disease" all correspond to leprosy and suggest Anglo-Saxon experience of it (4).

The fact that *likprar*, the Old Norse and Icelandic name for leprosy, is derived from the Anglo-Saxon *likprowere* (to suffer) implies that the Norsemen acquired both the name and disease from the British Isles before the Norman conquest. The eleventh-century Norwegian Gulathing's law relieved lepers (*likprar men*) from war-service. Disease plausibly interpreted as leprosy is mentioned in the Icelandic Bishops Sagas, which, although first written down about the thirteenth century, are of earlier origin (5).

If these records are insufficient to prove the existence of leprosy in the British Isles before the crusades, the foundation of leper hospitals before the first Englishmen sailed on a crusade in 1096 dispels all doubt. Archbishop Lanfranc, who died in 1089, founded the leper hospital of Harbledown near Canterbury during his lifetime. St. Leonard's hospital at Northampton was founded before 1087, and several others were founded before the turn of the century.

Attitudes towards lepers in medieval Europe shared a uniformity imposed by one Church. Only by understanding the reasons behind these attitudes can the full impact of the disease upon those who suffered from it be uncovered. Because the pattern of reaction to lepers was similar throughout the medieval world, those reactions can be examined almost as well in one country as another, but best perhaps in a country beside the mainstream, where, by virtue of relative isolation, traditions remained purer and lasted longer. There is no more suitable choice than Britain, where insularity and good documentation were happily combined. More representative attitudes are found in the countryside than in the towns, where disease, vagrancy, and disorder were often difficult to separate. The consequences of these medieval attitudes for individuals are most clearly seen later in Scandinavia during its slow emergence from the Middle Ages and thereafter.

Medieval leprosy has indelibly marked attitudes, language, and literature. The taunt of "moral leper", used recently even by a British Prime Minister, owes more to medieval tradition than to continuing experience of lepers as outcasts of society. Moral connotations of the disease can be traced through the sixteenth to nineteenth centuries in the imagery of phrases such as "ye lepre ... of ye saull", a "sinne leapered age", "lepered with so foule a guilt", "the Leprosie of Sin", "Leprosy'd with Scandal", and "leprosy of false knowlege" (6). William Cowper summarised his view of moral decadence in the lines:

> "When nations are to perish in their sins,
> 'Tis in the church the leprosy begins."

And in 1847, Tennyson wrote

> "A moral leper, I,
> To whom none spake."

Leprosy also appeared in terms of disgust and contempt. Coghill's rendering of Chaucer's "Canterbury Tales" has the Friar shunning the "scum of wretched lepers ... the slum-and-gutter dwellers" (7). Shakespeare prompts Margaret of Anjou to ask

> "Why dost thou turn away and hide thy face?
> I am no loathesome leper, look on me!"

And he describes the poison prepared for Hamlet's father as a "leperous distilment" which made his body "most lazar-like with vile and loathesome crust".

Medieval sermon and literature, in harmony with the contemporary image of the disease, portrayed leprosy as punishment meted out for moral failing, especially for loose, wanton, and lustful living. One work, the "Testament of Cresseid" by Robert Henryson (8), schoolmaster at Dunfermline in Scotland, is unique in its perceptive handling of a heroine's fall and leprous fate. Although the description of Cresseid's disease is traditional, Henryson's poem displays such feeling for the tragedy of the disease that it is hard to resist the conclusion that he had first-hand knowledge of lives broken by it, a credible inference because leprosy was still active in Scotland when he wrote.

Cresseid diagnosed her own disease, as many others must have done before and since, before sharing her secret with her father, who reacted with horror, sorrow, and despair:

> "He looked upon her ugly leper face,
> Which before was white as lily flower;
> Wringing his hands, he oftimes said alas
> That he had lived to see that woeful hour;
> For he knew well that there was no succour
> To her sickness, and that doubled his pain;
> Thus was there care enough between them both."

Recovering his composure, her father moved from resignation to resolution. Anxious to avoid the scandal of public diagnosis he took her secretly to "yone hospitall at the tounis end", equipped with "cop and clapper"—a bowl into which to receive her alms and a clapper to warn others of her coming.

Already her face was so disfigured that many people no longer recognised her:

> "Some knew her well, and some had no knowledge
> Of her because she was so deformed,
> With her face o'erspread with black boils,
> And her fair colour faded and altered.
> Yet they presumed because of her great distress
> And quiet mourning, that she was of noble kin;
> With better will they therefore took her in."

Her warm welcome in the leper house was more than deference to her high rank; doubtless the lepers anticipated a share in her subsistence while she lived and a handsome bequest when she died.

Hope had deserted her; position and comfort were lost; she had fallen captive to an incurable and fatal disease:

> "O sop of sorrow, sunken into care,
> O captive Cresseid, now and ever more
> Gone is your joy and all your happiness on earth;
> Now you are destitute of all joy;
> No medicine can heal or cure your disease!
> Your fortune is cruel and your fate is dreadful,
> Your joy is banished and your sorrow now sprouts."

Her suffering was not only mental but physical too, for her new surroundings were a far cry from her former comfort—

"Take this leper lodge for your lovely bower,
And for your bed take now a bundle of straw,
For choice wines and meats you once enjoyed
Take mouldy bread, perry, and cider sour.
Except for cup and clapper everything is gone."

But most tormenting of all her griefs was the ruin of her beauty. All that so recently had been seductive was now repulsive:

"My clear voice and courtly carrolling
With which I joined in singing with the ladies
Is hoarse as rook, full hideous, rough and raucous;
My pleasant bearing, all others surpassing,
Of lustiness I was held most worthy—
Now the appearance of my face is deformed;
No man now likes to look upon it.
Drowned in sorrow, I say with sore sighing,
Lodged amongst the leper people, 'Alas!'"

Alas, indeed, but horrid though her new companions may have seemed, one at least was not wanting in human kindness. A leper woman attempted to comfort her, and remonstrated kindly with her for fighting fruitlessly against her fate. Tears only deepened sorrow; better to make the best of a bad situation.

"Thus chiding with her sad destiny,
Weeping she lay awake throughout the night;
But all in vain; her sorrow, her careful cry,
Might not remedy, nor relieve her mourning.
A leper woman arose and went to her,
Saying, 'why do you kick against the wall
To kill yourself and mend nothing at all?

Since your weeping only doubles your woe,
I counsel you to make virtue of necessity;
Learn to clap your clapper to and fro,
And live according to the law of leper people.'
There was no remedy, so forth with them she went
From place to place, while cold and hunger sore
Compelled her to become an absolute beggar."

One of her first acts in the hospital, prompted doubtless by the rules of the house (see p. 163), was to compose her last will and testament. To worms and toads she consigned her corpse; to her companions she bequeathed the wealth they had coveted since she first stepped inside their door.

"When this was said, with paper she sat down,
And in this manner made her testament:
'Here I bequeath my body
With worms and toads to be rent;
My cup and clapper, and my ornament,

And all my gold the leper folk shall have,
For burying me in the grave when I am dead.' "

Cresseid's shattered aspirations, her disfigured body, her despair, and her inescapable death reflect truth far stranger than fiction, a reality which the experience of later centuries corroborates in the smallest detail.

Literature has preserved one part of the picture, folklore another. No simpler and more poignant memorial to the medieval leper exists than the chequered, bell-like fritillary, *Fritillaria meleagris* (Frontispiece). Around Crediton in Devon about one hundred years ago the triad of lepers, bells, and blotches lived on in the name of this delicate meadow flower, known locally as the "Lazarus bell" or "leopard lily" (9). Lazar was a medieval synonym for leper, and when, with the passing of the years, the spotted leper and his bell or clapper faded from popular memory, corruption of lazar into Lazarus (from which the name derived) was not surprising, nor was the corruption of leper into leopard an unreasonable attempt to preserve the image of the chequered spots; by that time, after all, leopards were no more exotic in Devonshire than lepers.

Use of the name lazar for leper is symptomatic of the deep confusion upon which the Church based its attitude towards leprosy and those who suffered from it. Lazarus, the beggar covered with sores, who in the parable lay at the rich man's gate, was apocryphally considered to have been a leper. An early English medieval example of this attribution is found in Aelred's prayer that the soul of David of Huntingdon, founder of a leper hospital, should be received "into the bosom of Abraham with Lazarus, whom he did not despise but cherished" (10). This unfounded attribution was widespread: many leper hospitals on the continent of Europe were dedicated to St. Lazarus; an order of chivalry, the Knights of St. Lazarus, separated from the Knights hospitallers in the late eleventh century to devote themselves (in theory if not in fact) to the welfare of lepers; hospitals for lepers were widely referred to as lazar-houses.

Lazarus, the unfounded leper, was only the beginning of confusion. By some strange and tortuous thinking, Lazarus the beggar became identified with Lazarus of Bethany, whom Jesus raised from the dead, conveniently perhaps, for it may have seemed to promise certain resurrection to the lepers. From this mistaken identity it was only a short step to link his sisters Mary and Martha with the welfare of lepers. Thus the Knights of St. Lazarus became known as the Knights of St. Lazarus and St. Mary of Jerusalem. Hospitals, such as the large and famous Sherburn hospital near Durham, were dedicated to "St. Lazarus and his sisters Mary and Martha". Even more curious was the fact that Lazarus soon vanished almost completely from England, leaving his sisters Mary and Martha, beatified, conjoined, and confused as St. Mary Magdalene, to protect most English medieval leper hospitals. In the vernacular, the leper hospital became the "Magdalene", "Mawdelyn" or "Maudlin", a name which still survived in 1880 in Totnes in Devon, where "Maudlin rentals" were collected by the corporation from lands which had belonged to the medieval leper hospital of St. Mary Magdalene of Totnes.

The final twist of the screw of patronal confusion came about when the more pragmatic Scandinavians saw in St. George and the dragon (Plate 1) the perfect allegory of the fight of the faithful against this disease. In Denmark, Sweden, Norway, and Finland, most leper hospitals were dedicated to St. George (Plate 2).

Only a handful were entrusted to St. Mary Magdalene including Viborg, the most eastern of them all near the border of Finland and Russia, a testimony probably to its large population of foreign merchants. Thus England lost her patron saint to the lepers of Scandinavia, whilst giving her own into the hands of a female and curiously mongrel saint.

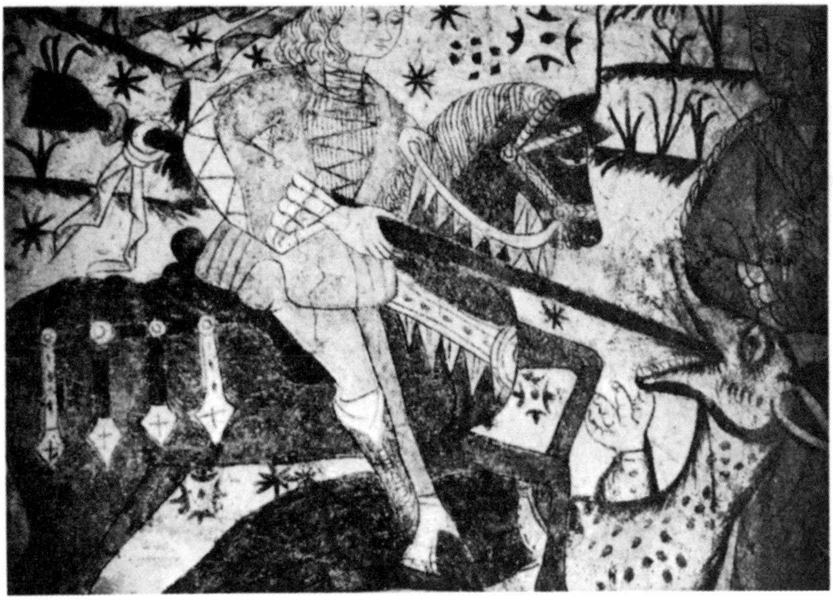

Plate 1. St. George and the dragon: detail from a medieval mural in Bellinge church, Denmark.

Patron saints were only one aspect of confusions compounded. Leper hospitals were placed outside the town, according to the Levitical precept that the leper should dwell "without the camp". The Church was right about Leviticus but wrong about the disease. As a result of translation through four languages, a diffuse Levitical concept of ritual defilement became identified with a disease answering to the description of modern leprosy. According to Levitical law, several ceremonially defiling conditions, including a disfiguring disorder of the skin summarised by the Hebrew word *tsara'ath*, necessitated separation from both the religious and secular communities; this word was translated into Greek as *lepra*. Leprosy, which Greek physicians described in unmistakable terms, was called *elefantiasis* on account of the elephantine appearance of the face deformed by excessive nodulation in the advanced disease. Greek medicine reached western Europe in Arabic translations but Arabic already had a disease, *das fil*, equivalent in name to *elefantiasis*. This tropical disease caused by filarial worms is still known as elephantiasis today, because limbs grossly swollen and wrinkled by the disease resemble elephants' legs. A different Arabic word, *juzam*, was therefore used to describe Greek *elefantiasis* (modern leprosy). *Juzam*, alas, was later translated into Latin as *lepra*, the same word as the Greek description of a vague collection of different diseases. At a stroke, a well-defined and specific disease of no religious significance was thus blurred into the diffuse Levitical concept of impurity.

In the fullness of time the Latin *lepra* and the equivalent English word leprosy, acquired all the religious overtones of the Hebrew *tsara'ath*. Medieval medical authors recognised the confusion and distinguished between "leprosy of the Greeks" and "leprosy of the Arabs", correctly identifying the latter with Greek

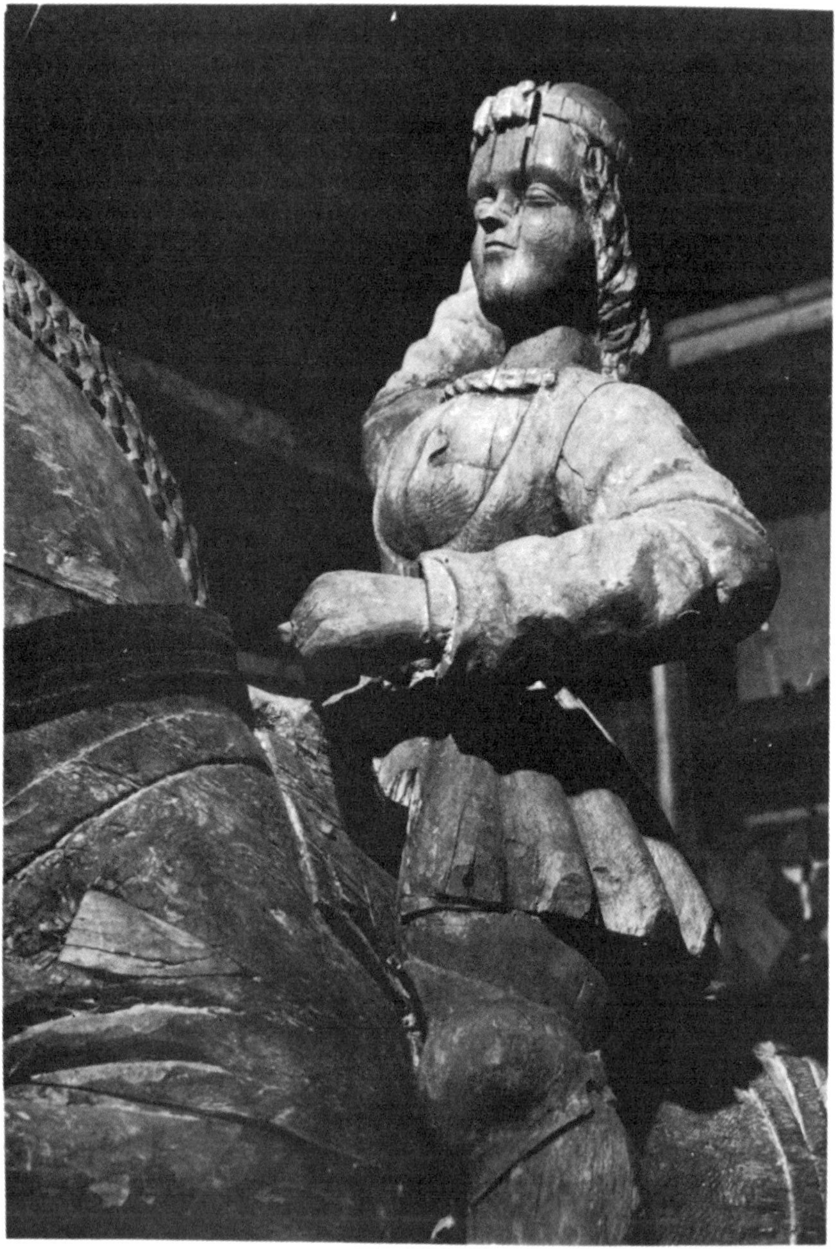

Plate 2. St. George: detail from a wood-carving in Hollola church, Finland.

elefantiasis and giving it the same title in Latin. Their insight was not shared by the Church.

It will never be known whether leprosy was sufficiently common in the early Middle Ages to justify the attention it received. Nothing in the foundation charters of the hospitals reveals an urgent concern to stem a flood of disease. Creighton may well have been correct in his surmise that lepers were never more numerous than village idiots (11). In their thirteenth- and fourteenth-century heyday there were about two hundred leper hospitals in Britain: they ranged from substantial ecclesiastical foundations, such as Harbledown near Canterbury and Sherburn near Durham, which housed 100 and 65 lepers respectively with a large staff of monks, to poor hovels without staff or chapel. Most hospitals originally had a chapel (many of which still exist in England), an administrator, a priest, and accommodation for about 10 lepers. No more than about two thousand British lepers are likely to have been in an institution at any one time out of a total population of about three millions; probably the number in hospital was soon substantially less.

The number of hospitals cannot be taken as a reliable indication of the prevalence of the disease. Early in the fourteenth century, when the number of foundations was at its peak, the disease was uncommon and declining. In 1344, four years before the Black Death reached England, St. Julian's hospital near St. Albans housed only two or three lepers, many fewer "than could adequately be sustained". Likewise, the early fourteenth-century revision of the regulations of Sherburn hospital allowed for the eventuality that there might not at any one time be a sufficient number of lepers in the diocese of Durham to fill the 65 places. When a place became vacant another leper from the diocese was to be admitted forthwith "if there are that many lepers there", otherwise the hospital authorities were to search further afield.

The mushrooming of leper hospitals in the early Middle Ages indicates that the disease was widespread, but it does not prove that leprosy was either common or increasing. Before inferring an explosive outburst of the disease it would be wise to ask why the hospitals were founded. Were they established to combat an epidemic or was there another reason? If these hospitals were primarily dedicated to the public health, why were the resources of some so curiously directed: St. Giles' leper hospital at Norwich, to take an extreme case, had an establishment of a master, 8 chaplains, 2 clerks-in-holy-orders, 7 choristers, 2 sisters, and 8 lepers; why not a master, a chaplain, 2 sisters, and many poor lepers?

It was a common medieval practice to set up a chantry chapel and to endow it for a priest, deacon, or (cheaper still) a clerk-in-holy-orders to say prayers and masses *in perpetuo* for one's soul. A more fashionable and impressive gesture, because of the special status the Church had mistakenly conferred upon leprosy, was to found a leper hospital, and thus to garner the fruits of both perpetual charity and perpetual prayer. Some of the smaller hospitals were little more than chantry chapels with an annex for lepers, such as St. Mary Magdalene at Taddiport near Little Torrington in north Devon, the chapel of which still stands, and which is referred to in contemporary documents as "*cantaria capelle Beate Marie Magdalene*". The great monastic foundations, such as St. Julian's near St. Albans, emphasised the achievement of God's greater glory, but did not entirely forget the souls of the benefactors; in the words of the regulations of the foundation its purpose was

> "... a deep desire for the glory and honour of our Lord Jesus Christ, His blessed Mother Mary, St. Alban, St. Julian and all God's saints and for the souls of King Offa and all our and the hospital's benefactors". (12)

Many benefactors made no apology for a business-like approach to their foundation. Robert de Roos founded Bolton hospital in Northumberland in 1225 "for the health of my soul and for all my predecessors and successors". The next year, Alexander II of Scotland founded Elgin hospital "for the love of charity, for the soul of King William, and for the salvation of my noble lord King Alexander". Cardiff leper hospital, a foundation of burgesses not royalty, was founded in the reign of Richard II

> "... for the good state of the King, the Earl of Gloucester, and the burgesses and commonalty, and for their souls after death, and to maintain 24 beds in the hospital for leprous, poor and feeble persons ...". (13)

Viborg hospital of St. Mary Magdalene on the marches of Russia was pragmatically founded by the governor of the castle "partly for the general welfare and partly to promote his own eternal happiness". In short, medieval leper hospitals were essentially the expression of charity engendered by a heavenly bandwagon, not a spirited defence of the national health.

Gifts were also made for a spiritual return. King Henry III in 1232 granted "for the health of his soul" a load of firewood daily to the lepers of Shrewsbury. Eight years previously he had issued a certificate to the Forrester of Shropshire, entitling the lepers of Bridgenorth to collect one horse-load of wood daily "for the reverence of God, and for the health of our soul and the soul of the lord King John". The spirit of charity in return for prayers outlasted the Middle Ages. In 1664 the lepers of Gloskär hospital on the Åland islands voiced their suspicion that they were not receiving the entire proceeds of the almsboxes placed in the harbours for their benefit; they quoted the servants of some who had contributed to the almsboxes as saying,

> "... if my master and mistress knew that the poor did not receive a penny they would not have given anything, for on account of these gifts the sick pray for those who give." (14)

Thus the wheel turns full circle back to the lepers of Åland.

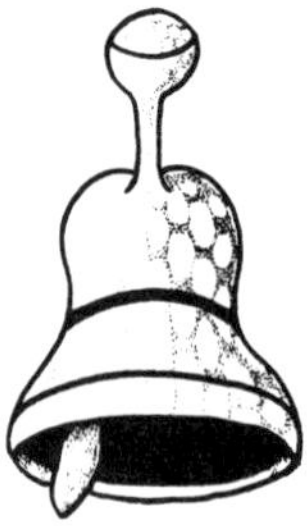

II

The Lepers of Åland

Of all the thousands of uninhabited islands in the Åland archipelago, one is unique. Gloskär (Lagoon Island) is half a mile long and a few hundred yards wide. Its surface, part bare outcrops of rock and part a dense, almost impenetrable thicket of pine, spruce, alder, and juniper, is deeply furrowed by inlets and ravines. On

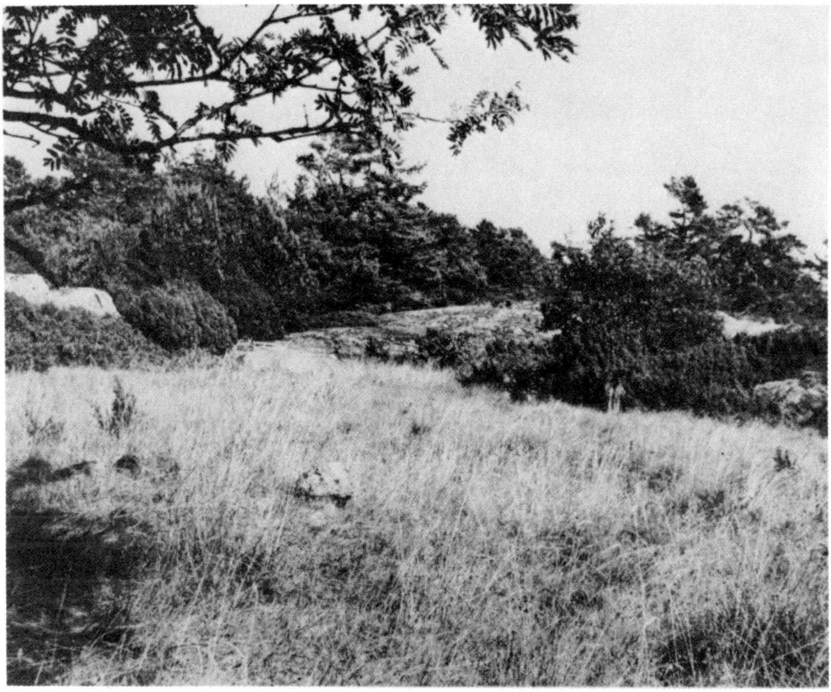

Plate 3. Site of the leper hospital on Gloskär, Åland islands.

the crest of the island, in its north-eastern corner, lies a T-shaped meadow, the only grassy plain on the island, and at that no longer than eighty yards. Two piles of jumbled boulders and the grass-covered foundation of a wall are today the only clues to its past.

This was not an island to covet in a sea of better islands. Doubtless for that very reason, this "small and lonely island ... near the village of Skogboda in the parish of Föglö" was on November 19th, 1651, chosen as the site of a hospital for the lepers of Åland (map and Plate 3). The order was signed by the governor-general of Finland himself, Count Per Brahe (Plate 4), a man whose concern for Finland so far exceeded the bounds of duty that his self-pronounced epitaph was

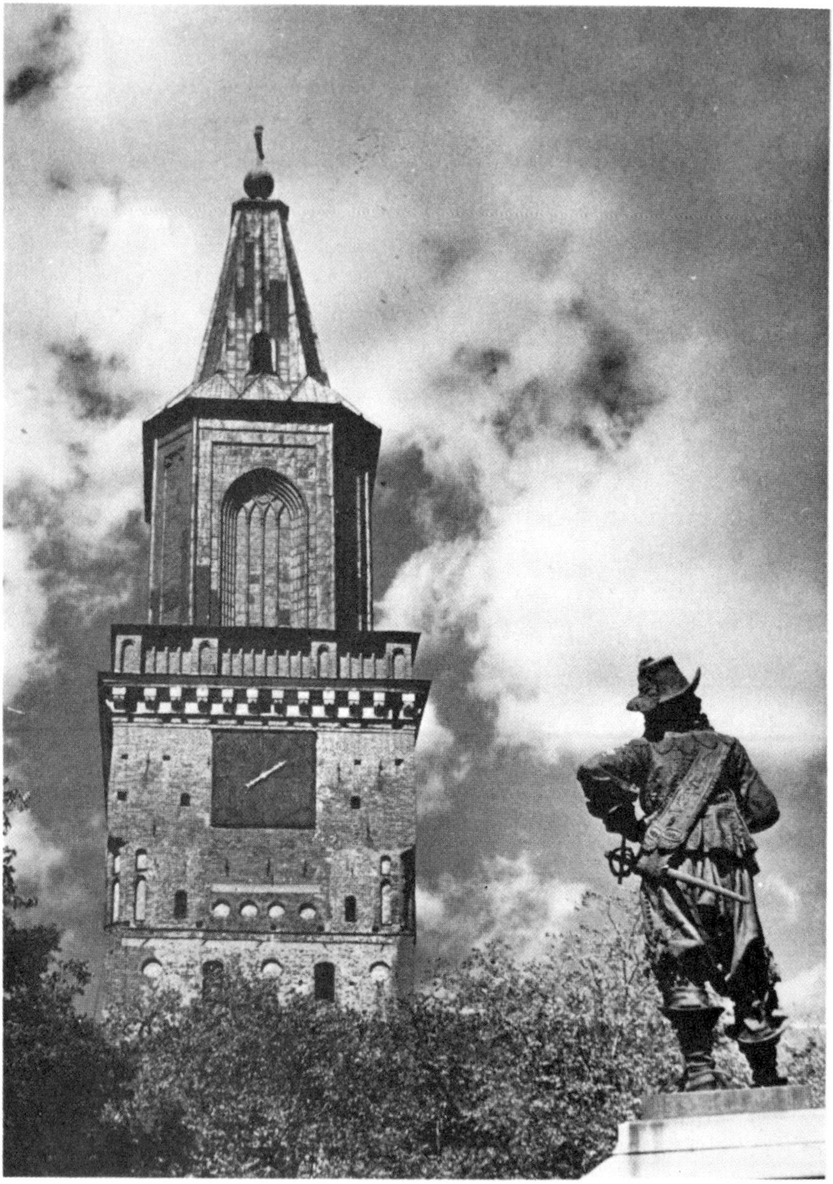

Plate 4. Statue of Per Brahe, Regent of Finland, by Åbo cathedral.

not contested: "I was highly satisfied with this country", he declared, "and this country with me."

A hospital on Gloskär was a victory (a somewhat pyrrhic victory in the event) for Boëtius Muur, rector of the parish of Saltvik (Plate 5) and dean of Åland, who for more than a decade had been troubled at the plight of lepers scattered throughout the island parishes. The law required that they should be sent to hospital when diagnosis was established, but the nearest hospital for lepers was fifty miles away by sea on the island of Själö in south-west Finland. These were long miles in an open boat; in winter the sea was frozen and impassable (Plate 6).

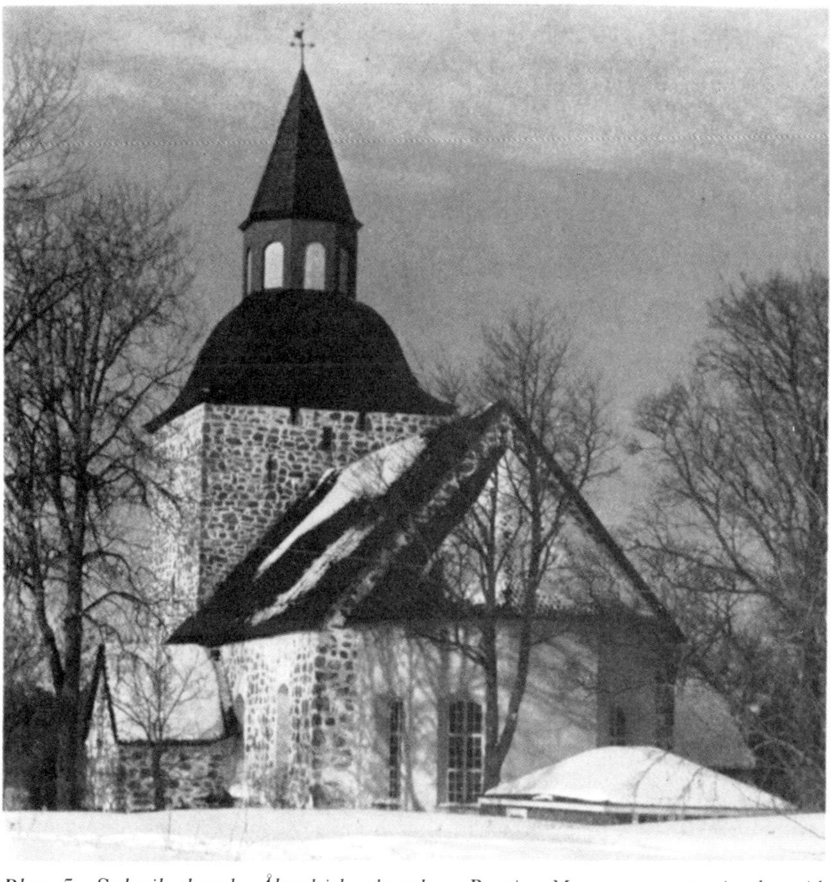

Plate 5. Saltvik church, Åland islands, where Boetius Muur was rector in the mid-seventeenth century.

On February 21st, 1648, Muur wrote to the cathedral chapter at Åbo, capital city of the Swedish province of Finland, suggesting that a hospital should be built on the Åland islands. He also asked them meanwhile to order the warden of the leper hospital at Själö to send a "large boat" to remove the lepers awaiting collection in the parishes of Åland. His personal requests to the warden had fallen upon deaf ears. "God knows", continued Muur, "how hard I find it to understand and to diminish this plague, which grows year by year in this country, in spite of the fact that many have been sent away, and many wise regulations have been made. If times were not so hard, it would not be necessary to ask the authorities to establish a hospital in this country."

A boat was eventually sent for the lepers, but communications did not improve and no hospital was founded. At a meeting of the parish of Hammarland on

January 27th, 1650, "the sheriff had to be reminded to remove the leper girl ... in the spring, after he had been reminded for several years". Three years after his approach to the cathedral chapter, Muur and the sheriff of Åland separately petitioned Per Brahe himself for a hospital. In November the count agreed, but not until August, 1653, was the hospital at Gloskär opened. It got off to a bad start, continued in misery, and ended in despair.

Per Brahe had not made any provision for a priest to serve the hospital, presuming, perhaps, that the rector of Föglö would automatically assume spiritual responsibility for the lepers. This omission caused a long and acrimonious dispute.

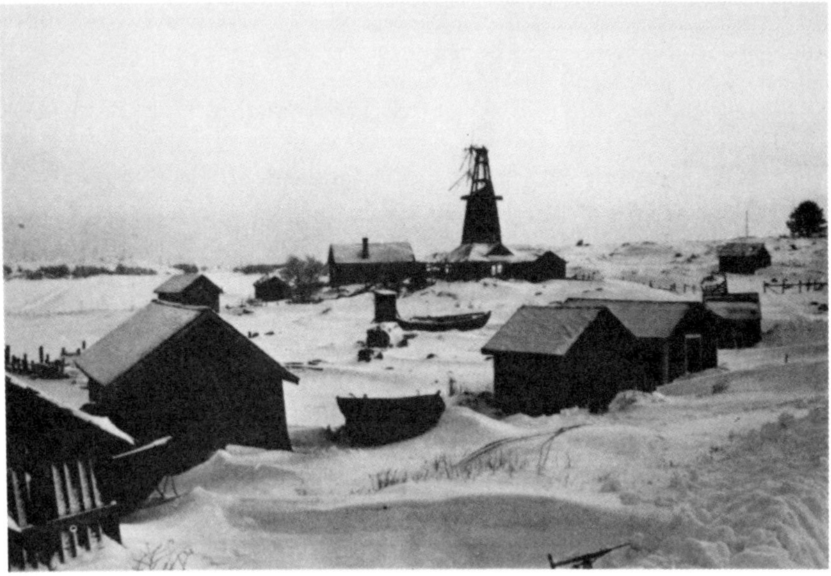

Plate 6. Åland islands in winter. This derelict scene on the edge of the frozen sea recaptures the atmosphere of Gloskär hospital.

In an isolated community, where the rector is nearer to God in power (if not in spirit), this mattered. The rector, Ericus Nicolai Nycopensis, flatly refused to countenance such a hospital in his parish. The record suggests that either laziness or fear made him unwilling to take the lepers under his wing. Possibly, however, he was under strong pressure from his parishioners to resist any such unwelcome and unhealthy incursion. His opposition was so successful that building was delayed. Eventually the authorities petitioned Per Brahe to admonish the truculent priest. In a letter from Stockholm dated July 1st, 1652, Brahe warned that "if the priest further objects to this or tries to prevent it, he will be severely reprimanded and summarily fined as punishment". These threats temporarily silenced the opposition, and building went ahead: two cabins for the lepers, a house a little distance away for the warden consisting of lobby, study and two other rooms, a sauna for the lepers, a cattle-byre, and a bake-house.

The parish priest was doubly defeated: Åland petitioned for separate support for a chaplain to the hospital. On June 21st, 1654, King Karl Gustav of Sweden graciously granted their request, making over for the use of a hospital chaplain one half of the parish tithe formerly received by the rector of Föglö. Ericus Nicolai grumbled at this injustice until his death in 1665; aggrieved and paranoid, he waged a ceaseless war against the inhabitants of Gloskär. How Lars Hammar, who was appointed both warden and chaplain to the hospital in 1654, fared personally in this war of attrition is not recorded, but so distraught was the rector of Föglö that in 1660 he petitioned the Swedish Parliament "with tears most humbly" for the return of the half of his church tithe diverted to the hospital chaplain to the "great harm and disadvantage" of both rector and parish (more, perhaps, to the detriment of the former than the latter). Alas for the rector in "his great need and poverty", his request was refused.

At about the same time, the rector of Föglö accused the hospital of interference with his fishing nets and the theft of one of his animals. On February 22nd, 1660, Muur investigated the complaint during his visit of inspection to Gloskär. Possibly theirs were crocodile tears, but Muur recorded that "it affected them deeply that they should have been suspected by Pastor Ehrich Nicolaj on account of the animal he has lost on one of his small islands". The fact of the matter was that, innocent or guilty, the rector was after their blood; Muur found it necessary to warn the lepers that if anyone of them ventured to set foot on someone else's island he "may freely be shot dead". The rector also complained that he had not caught any fish in neighbouring waters since the hospital was founded. He implied (not without foundation perhaps) that his nets had always been tampered with before his servants came to take them up. Muur did not pursue the matter; he simply "warned the sick in no way to misuse their boat, but to fish in the hospital waters, which are sufficiently extensive and full of fish". Perhaps to encourage them further in honest ways, he made sure on this occasion that they received the flax which they had requested for new nets.

If the rector of Föglö was living in straitened circumstances, so also was Lars Hammar, warden and chaplain to the hospital. Already in 1658 the total inadequacy of the hospital was revealed in the resolution of Muur's own parish of Saltvik that "lepers should not die of starvation, nor should they remain long in the parishes for the sake of being fed, which has been the situation for several years". The parishioners of Saltvik did not question the official plea that "the Crown is not in a position to contribute more in these times of war", but neither they nor the other parishes were better placed than the king. Income from alms dwindled to such an extent that the lepers became suspicious that they were being swindled. In 1664 Muur recorded their pointed request that "the money given by worthy gentlemen in the harbours should reach them".

In those difficult days rents were often not paid, and the parishioners were little short of mutinous in their poverty; indeed, they told their rectors to their faces that the population was decreasing, and they could not and would not contribute more. When people did make gifts it was both difficult and expensive to transport them between the islands. Uncertain communications partly account for the frequent complaints that the hospital received nothing on time from the sheriff. The difficulties in provisioning that lonely island in winter were indeed formidable: "Nothing can be done about the Christmas fare", Muur told the lepers in 1664, "because of the weather."

Whether because of hardship or neglect, the parishes gradually became less diligent in their duty to the hospital. Not only did they default on their customary Christmas gifts of food, but they often failed to ensure that new patients arrived at the hospital with the required food for their first few months there. In 1664

Muur reported that "the sick have not brought with them beer barrels, drinking vessels, . . . and several months' food according to the dean's order. It was decreed that the priest and church wardens should be fined if this instruction was ignored". More riot acts were read: for example, in 1665, "since Kumblinge parish send their lepers and have not given them Christmas food for more than one year, the sheriff is requested to use all means available to make them do their duty and show obedience". Haranguing had little effect.

All this was very disappointing, because great care had been taken to ensure the lepers' support. Casual charity was not enough, and the community was too poor to maintain regular payment of rents. Already in 1660, Muur had sent a dispirited report to the Swedish parliament, saying that the resources of the hospital at Gloskär were totally insufficient to clothe, feed, and house the lepers, who then numbered between twelve and sixteen. Others were still in outlying districts awaiting admission. The hospital, reported Muur, had only thirty daler left with which to buy food for the summer and nothing left over to pay for "even one stick of wood". Sadly, the man who had struggled so hard for the foundation of the hospital, and who had fought to sustain it, was forced to concede that the patients should be transferred to Själö in south-west Finland, where they had formerly been sent.

The king was decidedly displeased about the whole affair. A rather peevish reply was sent in his name on November 28th, 1660, saying that "The hospital, which was established on Åland a few years ago cannot be moved . . . just because of its difficulties. However, His Majesty will graciously consider how it can be provided with sufficient means to support the poor patients, when the official who is in charge of it gives a detailed explanation of why the means originally provided no longer suffice, and at the same time puts forward constructive proposals."

In his reply to this royal demand for an explanation, Lars Hammar attributed the destitution of the hospital to three major factors: first, embezzlement of part of the capital by the sheriff, Staphan Hansson, at the time of the hospital's foundation; second, an increase in the number of patients; and third, rising costs, particularly of firewood and boatmen's wages, the latter having recently doubled. Being more or less completely dependent on hired boatmen to transport their provisions, and not being a place that many boatmen would lightly visit, the hospital had to pay the market rate. The only benefit which the hospital obtained from this correspondence was a fixed annual income of two hundred daler from the revenues of Åland to replace various and uncertain rents received previously. That was an improvement, but it still was not enough.

Pastor Muur rowed, sailed, or sledged to Gloskär at least twice a year from 1658 to 1665, to inspect the conditions and to listen to the complaints of the patients and their warden. No matter was too small for his interest. One item only, the church services, was invariably to the entire satisfaction of the small community. Report after report opens with sentences such as "they have no complaints about God's word and the holy communion"—indeed they once reported that they had even had sermons on weekdays. It is always good strategy to preface a long list of complaints with at least one item of satisfaction.

Already in 1658, the two cabins for the lepers were falling down "from lack of care". They were repaired with the help of a gift of tiles and chalk from Saltvik parish, doubtless at Muur's instigation. In 1660, for the first and only time after the foundation of the hospital, it was reported that "all the houses are habitable".

But the hard winter took its toll; by the next summer Lars Hammar reported that his house was in disrepair and the two cabins lived in by the lepers were "very cold and without moss; daylight can be seen through the chinks and corners in many places". The lepers told Muur that the walls of one of their cabins were "rotten and would have fallen in long ago if supports had not been put against them"; it also lacked a covering of birch-bark or moss on the roof, and was so cold as to be declared uninhabitable. Thus both men and women were forced to huddle together for warmth in the other building, which itself "leaked in two places". This was hardly ideal accommodation for people suffering from a debilitating disease, in a winter cold enough to freeze the sea around their lonely island. The severity of the weather can be pictured vividly from the fact that "the cattle stalls had to be moved to higher ground, for in winter the cattle often walked in the snowdrifts on to the roofs of the sheds and trampled them to pieces".

By 1665 the situation was even worse. One shack was now completely abandoned and all the lepers lived in the other. Its gables were so drunk that "they did not know from hour to hour or from minute to minute when the roof will fall down and kill them". They might well have welcomed so swift a release from their sufferings. Not only were they threatened by the roof and exposed to the elements, but the floor was also disintegrating. Both grass-snakes and adders are common on the rocky, scrub-covered islands of the Åland archipelago, and panic gripped the lepers who now found themselves attacked not only by the elements from above and on all sides, but also from snakes below. Muur wrote that

> "the seven people who are still living ... have broken up all their chests and barrels to make a floor to walk on, because snakes crept in day and night and they did not dare all to sleep at the same time". (1)

The outbuildings too were in a state of decay. In the bakehouse, for example, "roof, walls and floor were all quite useless"—one wonders what was left.

The lepers hoped that the dilapidation of the hospital would persuade the authorities to rebuild it at a less godforsaken spot, "more convenient in-land where their families and other godfearing people could sometimes send them things". In this, as in so many other things, the miserable inmates were to be disappointed. In 1665, a new dwelling was erected for the lepers, who again possessed chests for their few possessions, for they requested that a large entrance hall should be added to the new building to house them. It should not, however, be assumed that the snake-fearing patients of 1664 had the means to acquire new chests to replace those broken up to make a floor. On the contrary, the likelihood is that these were new patients, because the turnover of patients was brisk: about one third of the little community died each year, and their number was replenished each spring and summer like a university replacing its graduates with new students. The bakehouse still had not been repaired, indeed besides needing new walls, roof, and floor, the oven itself was suffering from exposure and needed repair. The sauna was so decrepit that they had not dared to light a fire in it for six months; they had to wait another four years for a new one.

With such woefully inadequate accommodation it is surprising that anv of the inmates survived a single winter. The precise date of the death of only twenty-three of the lepers at Gloskär is recorded, and of these, eighteen died between November and April. The relative contributions of cold and malnutrition to their death is impossible to establish with certainty, but one clue suggests that malnutrition was the more important factor at neighbouring Själö in south-west Finland. Cold by itself would probably kill in January or February; malnutrition would tend to take its toll towards the end of winter. At Själö, where conditions were harsh, but not quite so severe as at Gloskär, the highest mortality was between March and May.

Although they regularly asked Muur for wool for stockings and linen for clothes, the Gloskär lepers never complained of being poorly clothed. Indeed, in July, 1665, they even stipulated that the six yards of linen which they needed should be "brown Holland"; perhaps the warden's wife had a hand in this request. For making shoes they asked for sealskin (unlike Själö, where cow-hide was requested), a reminder that seals were an important part of the economy of the Åland islands in the seventeenth century. Surprisingly seal meat is never mentioned as part of their diet.

Firewood was a more intractable need. In his petition for the foundation of a hospital on Åland, the sheriff, Staphan Hansson, had specifically mentioned fuel, asking that two loads of firewood should be contributed and delivered to the hospital by each parish—an important qualification when distances were long and across open water. To this request Per Brahe had magnanimously replied that

> "In so far as this does not affect the Crown, and the castle receives all the wood it needs, the aforementioned two loads of wood are granted to them with His Majesty's compliments, but only from the parish in which the hospital is built." (2)

Muur also raised the matter of firewood in his depressed report to king and parliament in 1660. The king's reply implies that none of the parishes was still under any obligation to provide wood for the castle, and as the wood for the hospital graciously granted by the Crown from the parish of Föglö was diverted from that due to the castle, the hospital could expect no wood by right. Because an earlier royal proclamation had relieved the Ålanders of their obligation to provide the Crown with wood, on account of the difficulty they had experienced in fulfilling their commitment, the king professed himself unable to force the parishes to supply wood to the hospital. With royal resourcefulness, however, he then suggested that persuasion might be tried:

> "However, His Majesty will graciously allow that if the hospital's means are insufficient, and no other way out can be found as far as firewood is concerned, then the sheriff must see whether he can persuade the parish of Lembland to provide the poor lepers with wood, because this is a Christian work and it is the duty of everyone to help the poor" (3)

—except the king?

Persuasion failed, for the parishioners knew their rights. The lepers told Muur in July, 1661, that "firewood has been scarce in recent years because many villages in Lembland have defaulted, some on their own initiative, some claiming old custom, and others on account of exemption granted". Lars Hammar elaborated, saying that "The hospital cannot expect any firewood from the parish of Lembland; in the past year and winter the hospital has suffered great hardship from cold and lack of wood for cooking, brewing, baking etc., and neither I nor the lepers can bear to stay at the hospital under these conditions any longer." Bear it or not, they had no alternative but to stay where they were, and they knew it.

Juniper bushes growing on the surrounding small islands were the only alternative fuel. On Muur's visit to the hospital in 1658 the lepers had requested permission to use the hospital boat to collect juniper bushes. As they denuded the nearest islands they had to search further and further afield, for "whereas junipers were hitherto plentiful on the outlying rocky islands none are now to be found". Their search for fuel as the winter of 1660/61 quickly closed in upon their island nearly ended in disaster. When Muur visited the hospital a few months later they told him the story:

> "The lepers complain with tears in their eyes that last autumn and winter they would surely all have died of cold if they had not gone out to the surrounding islands and pulled up juniper bushes. The ice was forming and they ran into great difficulties amongst the ice-floes, having to break up the ice all day long. Their boat would have gone down with its crew if they had not taken two other boats with them, which had brought lepers from the parishes." (4)

As it was, their boat was seriously damaged and they asked for a replacement. Firewood remained critically short, so short that in 1664 the warden indented for a new fence to replace his which the lepers had burnt for firewood.

The loss of the hospital boat in the ice-floes would have been a catastrophe for the little community. Muur often mentions the need to repair or replace the boat, which was used to ferry cattle from rough pasture to rough pasture on the outlying islands, to take one of the lepers to milk the cattle morning and evening in summer, and to fetch provisions, firewood, and hay from Föglö. Winter fodder was a serious problem, for they could not hope to grow sufficient hay on their small island. They requested the right to glean what they could, asking "if field hay and straw could graciously be left by Föglö parish, since other parishes in the country are far away, and it is difficult to transport it over such a long distance".

But if life would have been very difficult without their boat, it might have become impossible for those few left behind on the island if their able-bodied colleagues had perished with it. This was essentially a self-help community, usually numbering about ten persons altogether, some of whom would have been prevented by their disease from contributing their share of the work. Lars Hammar, who was both their administrator and comforter, farmed for himself in a small way, and probably took no part in their daily care. As both warden and chaplain he was in a difficult position: as warden he was strictly forbidden under Per Brahe's original regulations (5) to mix with the sick, either on the island, in their dwellings, on outlying farms (the small offshore islands), or in the church pews; but as priest he could not separate himself from his people. The command not to mix with them in the church pews was somewhat academic because they had no church, and it is most unlikely that the rector of Föglö would have had them in his, which in any case was miles away.

A brewer (perhaps a man from Föglö who visited from time to time) is the only outside helper mentioned, mentioned only to record that in 1664 Lars Hammar was no longer able to retain his services "for such small pay". Brewing for the lepers was a thankless task for they frequently complained about the quality of the beer. In desperation, the warden had already told Muur in 1661 that they could brew their own beer "because they seem to expect the same quality of drink whatever the quality of the harvest". Arrangements were also made for their grain to be milled for them, because "they have not sufficient strength to grind it themselves and they cannot live without it".

In spite of his relative independence, Lars Hammar could not insulate himself from the privations of his flock. The horror of the suffering and the strain of trying to save the small community from starvation or death from exposure fell heavily upon his shoulders. Muur came and went, but Hammar was there day after day, night after night. Muur had already reported in 1660 that the warden "longs for promotion from the hospital". As a compromise Hammar tried to obtain permission to live away from the island. The lepers, however, were most upset at this suggestion, rightly sensing no doubt that his constant presence was their only slender guarantee of survival. Thus "the sick asked Hr. Lars to remain on the island and on no account to move away to an untilled farm at Skogboda where he wants to live. However, they reluctantly suggested as an alternative, for the sake of peace, that the bishop should help to find them another chaplain and warden." But Hammar stayed, and there he died in 1667, his widow working out a "year of grace" by keeping the hospital accounts. She then moved to a nearby house with her six children and lived the rest of her life rent-free by royal dispensation. The new warden and chaplain was none other than Erik Portulinus, son of their old enemy, the rector of Föglö, who had died in 1665. Erik had tended the parish in his father's old age and illness, but had not succeeded to the rectorship on his death.

Five years later the utter destitution of Gloskär could be ignored no longer, and the hospital was closed. On August 12th, 1672, one of the saddest flotillas in the history of northern Europe set sail for the hospital on the island of Själö, fifty miles away. Twenty-three disfigured people with their pitifully few belongings were the only ugliness in a rippled blue sea, dotted with green and rocky islands, and bathed in soft autumn sunlight. The rippling of the water on the gunwales of their boats, the flapping of their rough sails, and the harsh shrieking farewells of the encircling gulls were the only sounds. One man and his family was left behind in the shambles of rotting shacks and scattered, jettisoned possessions. Erik Portulinus was chilled by the desolation of that lonely island more keenly than ever before. Grotesque and horrible his flock may have been, but they were a company of just-living people, and he had been their pastor and friend. Now he and his were the only living human flotsam on the deserted island; their company the cattle, the gulls, and the bones of eighteen years of human suffering locked in the shallow earth of a graveyard "packed so full that they could not bury any more corpses there".

Erik Portulinus had received scant reward for his five years of faithful service. For the first year, as the custom was, he had had to support his predecessor's widow. Now, the moment that the lepers' boats disappeared into the blue haze of the horizon, his salary ceased and he had only his small private means to exist on. Life had treated him hard. Some years ago he had lost "twenty cattle big and small, and two horses". Recently "God help us", he had lost "one horse, three oxen and nineteen old sheep" and, to crown it all, the farm in Åbo, which he had inherited from his wife's family, had been destroyed by fire. Exhausted and broken, he concluded "I have met with many more adversities too numerous to mention" and now "I no longer have the strength to live with these my poor ones".

His spirit may not have recovered, but he lived on. A royal warrant of December 13th, 1672, asked the bishop and chapter of Åbo cathedral to find a new living for him, but none was found. The problem, they said, was that he was unable to speak Finnish and no living in a Swedish-speaking community was vacant. Finland, then as now, was a bilingual country, with most of the Swedish-speaking minority living in Åland, west, and south-west Finland. It was a good excuse, but the real reason probably was that no parish would accept as pastor a man who had lived at close quarters with lepers for five years. Two years later Erik Portulinus was still marooned on his now-forgotten island. In a pathetic petition to the king of Sweden, he explained that "because of the strong and evil stench and odour of the lepers, I had to carry out my service in frost and cold, in sleet and rain, under the open sky. In autumn and spring I was often trapped in the sea-ice. Thus I have now become, God help me, an ailing man." He went on to describe how "in the greatest poverty I have to support myself, my poor wife and many small children ..." In spite of it all he lived on to die at the age of 71, twenty-three years later, as perpetual curate of Kökar, an outlying island whence many of the lepers had come.

The Gloskär lepers themselves also caused an ecclesiastical headache. The community of Själö hospital, where they now found themselves in the company of about forty other lepers, and within a stone's throw of about twenty mad or simple people, was Finnish-speaking. Their chaplain now had thrust upon him these twenty-three Swedish-speaking people who understood little or no Finnish. He at least, unlike the unhappy Erik Portulinus, was bilingual, but he complained bitterly to the Governor of Åbo that his work had doubled: he now must deliver his Sunday sermons and say prayers on Sundays and throughout the week first in one language and then in the other. With laudable pragmatism the bishop doubled his stipend.

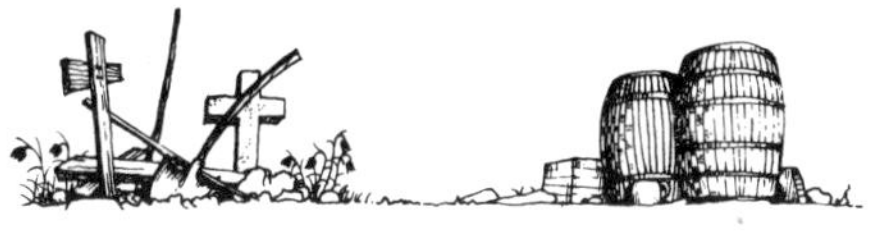

III

Bread, Beer and Firewood

Do the miserable conditions at Gloskär really represent the sufferings of lepers elsewhere in Europe at that time, or indeed at any other time? Extreme the privations certainly were, but they differed only in degree and not in kind from the hardships in other places and at other times. Climate and war made the latter half of the seventeenth century as hard for the North as any period, but the next two centuries were little easier. Leprosy is essentially a disease of the poor, and neither those who suffered from it nor the communities who supported them became more prosperous for a very long time.

Gloskär hospital itself was founded at a particularly bad moment in time. From 1655 (two years after the hospital opened) until 1660, Sweden under King Charles X Gustavus was continuously, expensively and often triumphantly at war; at first with Poland and her allies, and later with Denmark. Finland contributed heavily to the Swedish war-effort in both money and men. From that time until the end of the Napoleonic wars the resources of Sweden/Finland and of Denmark/Norway were frittered away in war. Further, their trade was recurrently interrupted both by their own involvements and by the wider ripples of European conflict.

In the seventeenth century abnormally cold weather compounded the misery. It was a century of continental climate throughout Europe, the hardest consequences of which fell upon the North. Not only were the winters colder, but they were longer; spring arrived late and autumn frosts set in before the crops were ripe. In 1696 Finland's harvest was ruined by early frost. When corn supplies were exhausted, the cattle were slaughtered. Then bread was made from pine bark and, finally, roots and chaff were eaten. One third of the population died from starvation or disease before the harvest of 1697 ripened, a mortality greater than during the Black Death in western Europe three and a half centuries earlier (1).

To a large extent, therefore, the hardships endured by lepers only mirrored the circumstances of the general population. Inevitably, in hard times, the weak, sick, and dependent suffer most. Those who look after them are not immune from their suffering. The warden and chaplain of Kronoby hospital, near Vaasa on the west coast of Finland, received so little of his stipend that in 1658 he took in kind what he was owed in cash. Three years later he was forbidden to do this; instead, his stipend was paid, leaving him much worse off because he had to buy his food out of a fixed income at a soaring market price. By 1667 he was so destitute that he was admitted as a pauper to his own hospital.

In times of hardship the administrator had to bear the brunt of the lepers' complaints: another warden of Kronoby hospital was accused of embezzling corn, butter, fish, and money belonging to the hospital in the famine year of 1696. The lepers threatened him with a law which stated that anyone guilty of stealing goods belonging to the poor, to a hospital, or to a church should be "sentenced with double the penalty imposed upon a common thief". The accused administrator rejected their charges with the sad comment "What is harder than to be house-keeper of an empty storehouse?"

Finland suffered most from the Scandinavian wars, not least because she was the buffer-zone on the long border with Russia. When Charles XII of Sweden met his match in Peter the Great, it was Finland that Russia invaded. The chaplain of Viborg leper hospital was so poor that when he fled from the front-line fighting in 1711 he only managed to support himself by pawning the hospital's communion cup. His flock vanished into the surrounding countryside; the hospital was burnt to the ground. By 1714 Finland was occupied by Russian troops. Those inmates capable of escaping from Själö hospital in the south-west corner of the country had fled. The chaplain abandoned the few who remained and made his escape to Sweden, taking with him the bells of the hospital chapel (whether for their safety or his own support is not clear), "which he moved from one place to another not without difficulty and expense". The hospital was pillaged by a dragoon despatched by captain Arkot, commander of the Russian occupation force in Åbo. His orders were to dismantle and remove to Åbo any wooden buildings serviceable for the Russian forces. It must have been one of the rare moments when the hospital was in good repair, for only one of the buildings was rejected out of hand. The local people were forced to pull down several houses and outbuildings, including the best house used by the lepers. Perhaps the lepers had the last laugh, picturing the Russian soldiers occupying their leprous quarters in blissful ignorance of their former use.

Living conditions for the population in general and the lepers in particular continued to be hard well into the nineteenth century. Even in Bergen, second city of Norway, the leper hospital was no better than medieval, and possibly worse. Here, in 1801, the unenviable post of chaplain to St. George's leper hospital (Plate 7) was taken by a young man, Johan Andreas Welhaven (Plate 8), a few months after he obtained his theology degree at Bergen university. To this task he devoted all but the last few months of his life; he died in 1828. Welhaven recorded in 1816 that the lepers lived in one long, narrow building containing a common living-room and forty rooms on two floors, rooms which were so small that there was barely room "for two people to turn around". Welhaven suppressed, but never completely overcame, his horror of the place:

> "Because of the exhalation from the patients the air in these narrow rooms is highly unhealthy, as I often experienced with loathing when I was called to my duties, or when my visiting in the parish brought me to the bed-ridden leper, particularly early in the day. This is even the case with the large room or hall of the hospital where all the patients undertake their daily work together. So many are collected together in the one place that the atmosphere soon becomes fouled by the many stinking breaths, and the food, which is consumed by everyone in that room and warmed on the stove in winter before meals, is also poisoned by it." (2)

The income of the hospital was inadequate for its needs: "The weekly allowance", wrote Welhaven, "is utterly insufficient for the lepers, therefore I find the constant

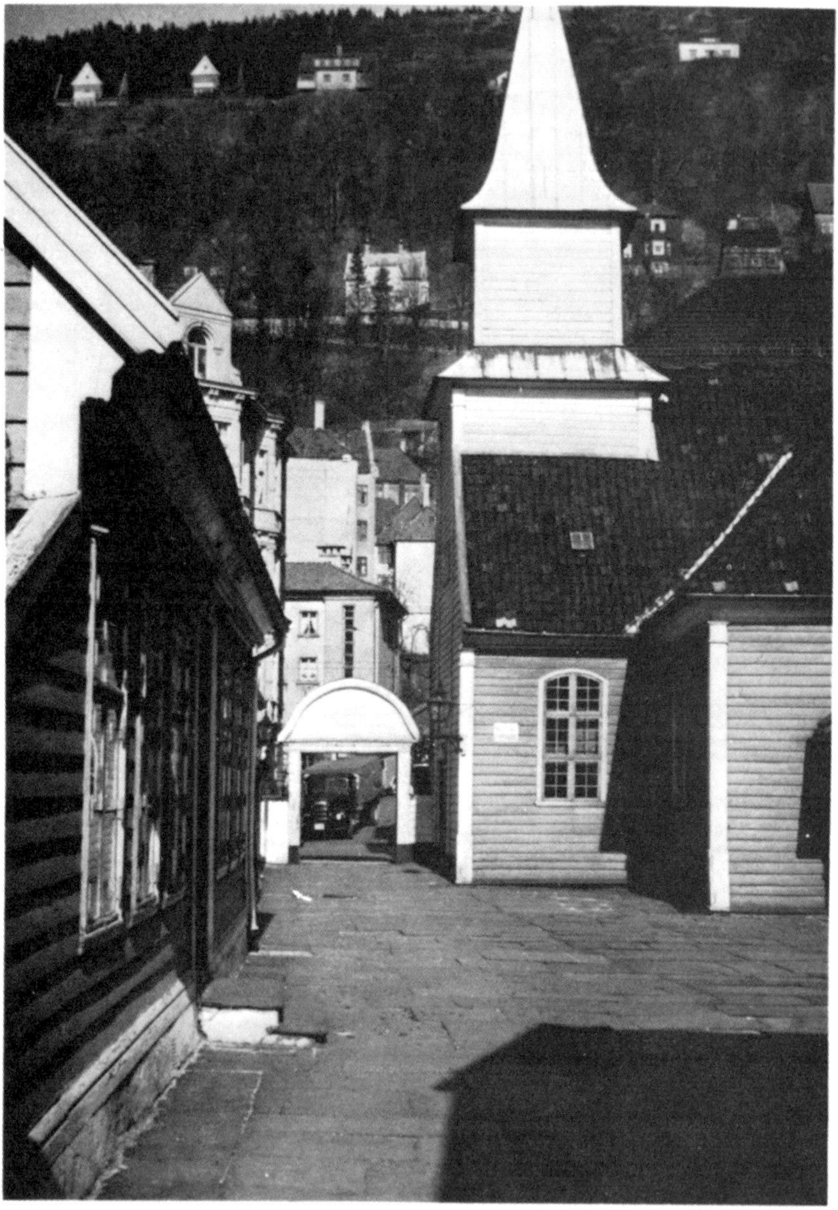

Plate 7a. St. George's hospital for lepers, Bergen. Founded in the Middle Ages, it was rebuilt in 1702 and enlarged in 1742 and 1857. It was closed in the 1920s but has recently been made into a leprosy museum.

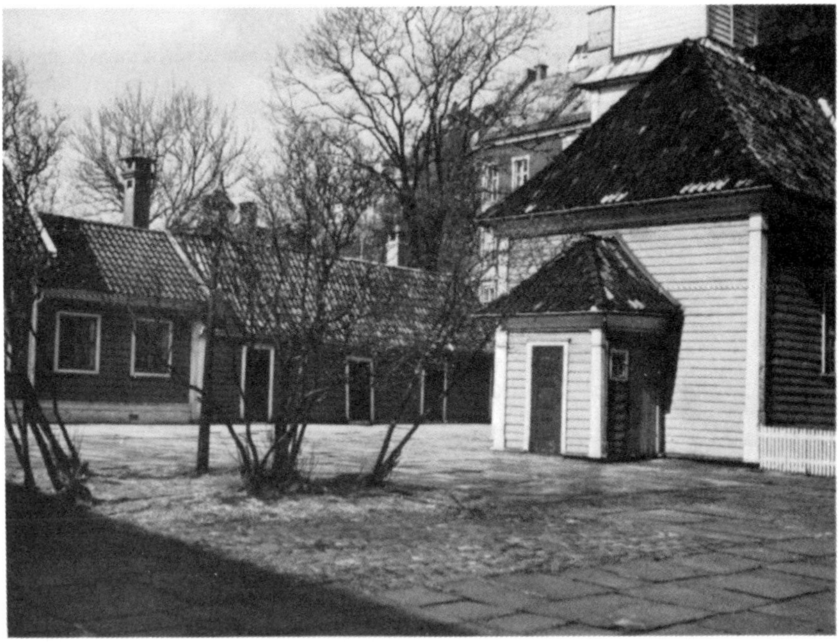

Plate 7b. St. George's hospital for lepers, Bergen.

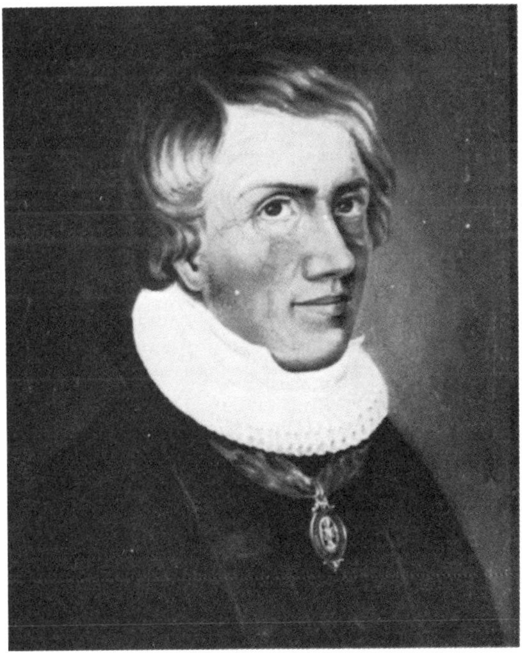

Plate 8. Johan Andreas Welhaven (1775–1828), chaplain of St. George's hospital for lepers at Bergen from 1801 to 1827, painted by his son Johan Sebastian Welhaven.

wish of these wretched people for more generous provision exceedingly reasonable." They were well satisfied with their customary diet of fish, bread, gruel, and milk, he said, "when they get enough", but he recalled that "during the former days of war fish was their only nourishment and life saving food, apart from a few crumbs of bread . . ."

This chorus of privation is a far cry from the letter of the regulations at the great medieval monastic foundations (3), where bread and beer were prescribed in plenty. Both St. Julian's hospital near St. Albans and Sherburn hospital (Plate 9) provided seven loaves per person each week; the Sherburn regulations, which

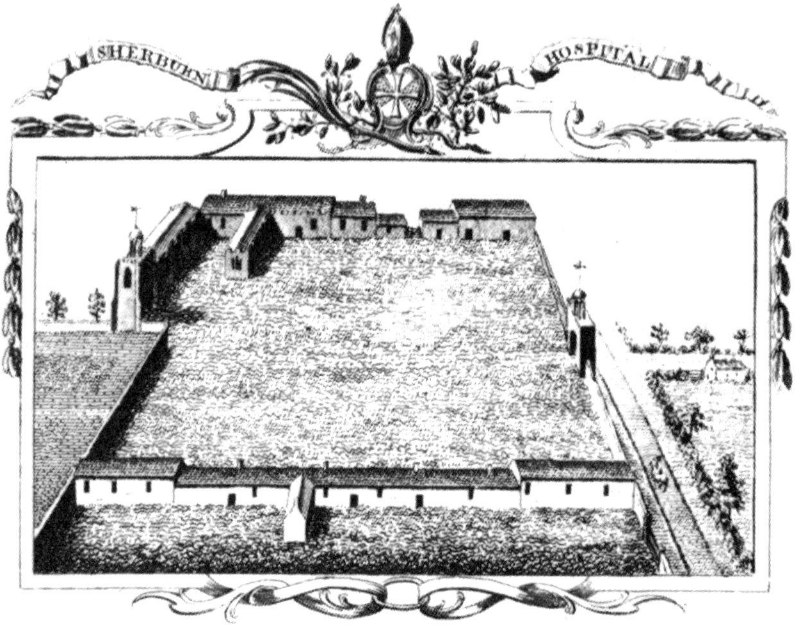

Plate 9. Sherburn hospital near Durham in the eighteenth century. Founded in 1146, the hospital became an almshouse in the sixteenth century when lepers could no longer be found.

had a greater air of reality about them, defined the weight of the loaves as five marks. Surprisingly, five of the seven loaves at St. Julian's were to be white, a stipulation which seems curiously out of tune with the ordinary diet of the time. Fourteen barley loaves per week were prescribed at Enköping leper hospital in Sweden, but the weight was not stated. Certain church festivals and saint's days merited an extra loaf: St. Julian's and Enköping hospital agreed that the festivals of the Virgin Mary and St. John the Baptist deserved a bonus—one loaf at St. Julian's and three at Enköping, but apart from those two days and the festivals of Christmas, Easter, and Whitsun, they celebrated different occasions with extra rations. In addition, Sundays at St. Julian's were regularly allocated an extra ten white loaves, five to be shared between the brothers and five amongst the sisters, preference to be given to the weakest.

Differences between the bread allowances at St. Julian's, Sherburn, and Enköping were small in comparison with variations in the authorised beer ration. The standard weekly ration was fourteen gallons (*lagena*) per person at St. Julian's, or eight pence in lieu, seven at Sherburn, and seven shared between five to eight persons at Enköping. Special festivals were celebrated at St. Julian's with a jar (*obbata*) apiece, or one penny *in lieu*, and by a gallon between twenty persons at Enköping; St. Julian's finally excelled itself with a veritable torrent of good cheer at Christmas to the extent of forty gallons apiece, or forty pence *in lieu*. By arrangement with one's colleagues one could clearly be both jolly and rich at St. Julian's at Christmas.

Curiously, the only mention of meat in the food regulations of St. Julian's is one pig per person at Martinmas, or money *in lieu*. Martinmas at St. Julian's conjures up a delightful picture of porcine and leprous revelry. The regulations required that the pigs were to be presented personally to the lepers "if it can conveniently be done", so that each in order of seniority should choose his own animal. Potherbs were provided in anticipation. Salt was distributed at St. Julian's once a year in the substantial quantity of two bushels per person. Sherburn provided salt whenever fresh meat, egg or fish was served; at Enköping salt was issued at Michaelmas, Easter, and the festival of St. John the Baptist.

Of the regulations of these three great monastic foundations those of Sherburn pay the most attention to everyday detail. Meat was, if possible, to be served on three days each week and fish on four; eggs were permitted as an alternative to fish. Butter and cheese were also approved alternatives to meat when "in season", an indication that milk output was not maintained throughout the winter. On special festivals both fish and meat were allowed. The most appetising festivals were Quadragesima, on which fresh salmon and "beans for roasting" were on the menu, and Michaelmas, when a goose was to be shared between every four persons with apples provided—the first documented appearance of roast goose and apple-sauce perhaps. The custom of the Michaelmas goose has disappeared from England, but continues in Denmark. Smoked beef is the only meat mentioned at Enköping. Surprisingly, the Enköping regulations permitted milk foods in Lent if fish were unobtainable. Can it really be that milk was more plentiful than fish in the south of Sweden as the long winter ebbed, or is this an inappropriate remnant of an archetypal regulation which originated in southern Europe? Fish doubtless was the protein of Lent and fast days in all hospitals. Occasionally the amount is specified, as for example the basic Lenten ration of one barley loaf, one wheaten loaf, and two herrings daily at Enköping, with a further fifty cod, fifty dried pike, two smoked salmon, and a bushel of peas to be shared between all the inmates during Lent. The tradition of fast days outlived the Reformation in Sweden and Finland; the opportunity to save food was too tempting to neglect. In the records of food provided at St. George's hospital in Åbo from 1558 to 1559, Fridays are omitted entirely. By 1598, Friday at least figured on the weekly menu, but only to be accompanied by the one word *intet*—"nothing".

Fifty years later, at Gloskär, fasting was dictated by shortage, not by the church calendar. The chance of obtaining anything other than fish and bread on that remote island for most of the year was small indeed, apart from the meagre milk of their two cows. But the medieval custom of extra allowances on special festivals had not been forgotten (4): on July 27th, 1661, the Gloskär lepers humbly requested "better drink and fresh meat at the festivals of Christmas, Easter, and Whitsun", a theme to which they returned three years later when they again begged to "refresh themselves with better food on the three festivals than they receive daily, both food and drink, which was the practice for some years and now has been discontinued".

Firewood was almost as essential as food, and this too featured in the regulations of the most prosperous hospitals. St. Julian's provided fourteen shillings to be shared between the brothers at Christmas to buy their fuel for the year, "as had been ordained of old for the sake of peace and concord". The lepers of Sherburn hospital were warmed at Christmas by four large tree-trunks, each "large enough for a cart in itself". For much of the year they warmed themselves with peat fires: in summer, they received the broken fragments of peat during cutting; in the autumn, two baskets of peat daily; and in winter, four baskets daily. Thomas à Becket, when Archbishop of Canterbury, allowed the lepers of Harbledown a one-horse cart to fetch wood daily from a neighbouring wood. So important was fuel that at Svendborg in Denmark their forest resources were carefully husbanded: the warden was forbidden "to fell trees, or to let others fell trees or spoil the woods belonging to the hospital". Important though firewood was in Britain and Denmark, nowhere was it more essential than in Finland, where it was a continually recurring theme both in hospital regulations and in the lepers' complaints.

Those medieval hospitals which insisted on a particular uniform (and probably only the biggest and best did) were expected to provide the cloth for it. Sherburn lepers were entitled to six feet of woollen cloth of white or russet colour, twelve feet of linen and twelve feet of canvas. Both at Reading and at Enköping twelve feet of cloth were due annually to each inmate. Money was given at St. Julian's for the purchase of shoes, and at Enköping two pairs were provided each year per person, one at Christmas and the other at the feast of John the Baptist. At Åbo in Finland, the lepers of St. George's hospital also received two pairs of shoes annually; in fact it was probably the rule in Scandinavia rather than the exception for the institution to provide shoes, the one important and expensive item of dress beyond the means of many men and women. Shoes also comprised part of the salary of the servants of St. George's hospital in Åbo in the sixteenth century, a custom which survived long afterwards at Själö hospital, where the four farm-workers each received one half of a "slaughter-cow" for meat and shoeleather.

Few lepers lived long enough to wear out the garments they brought to hospital, and probably for that reason clothes do not figure prominently either in provisions or complaints. At Gloskär those who lived long enough to become threadbare received wool, homespun cloth, and occasionally linen. Later, at Själö, some servants were paid partly in shirts and in wool for gloves and stockings.

Well-endowed monastic foundations were the exception, even in the early Middle Ages. Most leper hospitals were small, housing fewer than ten lepers, and their income was both small and uncertain. Within two centuries of their opening even the grandest were unable to fulfil their regulations. Both maladministration and national economic decline contributed to their reduced circumstances. Already in 1344, five years before the Black Death shattered the economy of Europe and claimed his own life, Abbot Michael of St. Albans stated that the endowments of St. Julian's hospital, a daughter foundation of his abbey, had been "diverted to unworthy and damnable uses, and were embezzled by usurpers". He probably referred to two of his predecessors: one was warned by the Pope in 1223 not to oppress the leper women at the sister foundation of St. Mary's; the other was accused in Chancery proceedings of oppressing the brethren of St. Julian's. In the north of England, at Sherburn hospital, the situation was no better.

IV

Means of Support

Throughout medieval Europe admission fees, gifts, tolls, and taxes helped to support leper hospitals, although their wealth depended mainly upon endowments. Their means also varied according to the expertise and integrity of their wardens, and upon the economic fortunes of the day. For a long time, fees paid on admission contributed little to the funds because lepers were poor, and what they could not pay was not paid.

Neither the regulations of Sherburn hospital nor those of St. Julian's refer to an admission fee, probably because both were unusually well-endowed. Admission fees certainly were expected at some leper hospitals in England: at Dover and in London a sum of one hundred shillings is mentioned, an amount far beyond the means of most lepers; an additional half mark was expected both by the warden and by the brothers as a sweetener from the new arrival. Fear of the disease was not sufficiently great to prevent some who were not lepers seeking food and shelter for their old age or infirmity in a leper hospital. The warden was thus sometimes tempted to admit the wealthy, who simply wished to be looked after and were prepared to pay for it, in preference to the poor lepers. This fact explains why, in 1303, admission to the hospital of St. Nicholas in York was forbidden "by agreement for money or goods". A visiting jury had discovered that many had been admitted in return for a fee of "20 marks, more or less". A healthy man was admitted to the leper hospital of St. Bartholomew in Oxford in 1321 contrary to the rules but by express command of the king, because he promised to pay for the repair of the roof of the hospital chapel. Danish leper hospitals also demanded an admission payment: St. George's hospital at Svendborg expected new entrants either to provide an endowment or to pay an admission fee, if it were within their means.

Seventeenth-century Finland continued the medieval tradition of an admission fee. Now, however, the parish was held responsible for whatever the leper and his family were unable to pay. No longer was the contribution of the parish limited to Christian charity. Assessment by the parish meeting of a leper's means became as important as the examination of his body. On February 7th, 1650, Pastor Muur reminded the parish of Lemland that after a person was formally declared a leper the parish priest should be notified whether or not he could raise the statutory admission fee. Later that year a meeting of the parish of Föglö was told that a leper boy from Hasterboda had been provided with the necessary fee, and the sheriff was thereupon asked to have him moved to hospital. Sometimes the admission fee proved too much, not only for the leper and his relatives, but also for the parish itself. The outlying island parish of Kökar was too poor to provide the fee for a leper girl in 1649. The problem was only solved by the church authorities taking twenty daler out of the "wreck money".

Seven years earlier, Bishop John Petri of Lindköping had petitioned the chancellor of Sweden for a reduction in the hospital admission fee which, he said, evoked "a great sigh from the people". Bishop Rothovius complained in 1643 that there were so many lepers in the archipelago of Åland and south-west Finland that "the parishes are unable to provide for them according to the hospital rules". Leprosy was pocketed in a few parishes: for some, such as Kimito near Åbo, which sent about fifty lepers to Själö in the first century of that hospital's existence, the financial burden upon the sparse population was heavy. Many entries in the Kimito parish records between 1623 and 1670 refer to sums paid to make up hospital admission fees for leprous parishioners. In 1682 each household in the parish was required to contribute 2 öre (32 öre = 1 daler) for a leper; in the year 1686/87 a total of 122 daler 30 öre of copper coin was collected for leper admission fees.

Twenty silver daler (1) was a substantial sum for small farmers and fishermen to raise. Even in 1695, after years of sporadic war and progressive inflation, it was still a considerable amount judged from the fact that the total value of the annual salary of the chaplain of Själö hospital in money and kind was 200 silver daler and the value of the warden's salary was 165 daler (2). At the other end of the scale, and much more to the point, the annual value of the farm-hands' allowances was 14 daler, the house boys' 8 daler, and the serving girls' only 5 daler. Corn cost $2\frac{1}{2}$ daler per tun, half a "slaughter-cow" cost 2 daler, 12 lbs of butter and 80 lbs of herring each cost 1 daler. Two shirts cost $1\frac{1}{4}$ daler and 3 lbs of wool for socks and gloves cost $\frac{1}{2}$ daler. The total cost of the annual food allowance for one person at Själö from 1695 until the regulations were revised in 1814 was just under 20 daler.

Throughout the Middle Ages, and for years afterwards, all entrants were expected to bring their everyday possessions with them—all their "moveable possessions", as the Enköping hospital regulations put it. The medieval church service for the seclusion of a leper (3) stipulated that besides clothes and "his signal the clappers", he should have sheets, crockery, cutlery, couch, coverlets, pillows, chest, table, candlestick, shovel, pot, and "other needful articles". In this obligation the leper was no different from his healthy but poor brother in an almshouse: for example, the fifteenth-century foundation of St. John at Heytesbury in Wiltshire required

> "that every poreman in his first admission all such moveable goodes as he hath, pottis, pannys, pewter vessel, beddyng, and other necessaries, if he have eny such thynges, to bryng hit within the hous". (4)

The regulations for Gloskär hospital in 1653 echo these medieval requirements, insisting that the lepers must bring with them cooking utensils, bedding and everyday clothes. It was up to the parishes to see that they complied. On March 13th, 1655, for example, at a meeting of the parish of Lemland, Kirsten of Söderby was instructed to take with her "cooking utensils, barrels, axe, grindstone or small whetstone, and sieve".

Much of the income of medieval hospitals was received in kind. The members of St. George's hospital at Svendborg, for example, received "corn, butter, money, lambs, geese, hens, and pannage" as dues from their estates. Between 1578 and

1612, Åbo castle delivered at Christmas and Easter a gift of bread, beer, ham, meat, fish, and hares to the town's St. George's hospital. Surplus quantities of any one item were sold, and the proceeds were used to buy other necessities. For this reason, and because inmates rarely received their full rations, any attempt to evaluate the nutritional value of the lepers' food from their official allowances at any period before the mid-nineteenth century is valueless.

Other dues in kind were received through a variety of local customs. By a privilege conferred by King John in 1204, the lepers of Shrewsbury were due a handful of corn or flour from sacks exposed at the market, and by order of the Earl of Chester the lepers of Chester were entitled to a toll on salt, fish, grain, malt, fruit, and vegetables at the market, as well as to one cheese or salmon from each load, and to one horse at the horse fair. The leper hospital at Carlisle received several sheaves of corn from each carucate of land in Cumberland; a similar tax was paid by farms in the Durham bishopric to Kepier leper hospital. Carlisle lepers were also granted by the mayor and citizens a "pottle" of ale from each brew-house and a farthing loaf from every baker who displayed his bread on Sunday. In 1443, bakers who baked underweight loaves, or who in other respects failed to observe the law, were ordered to forfeit their bread to the leper hospital in Copenhagen. Not only food sold unlawfully, but also food too rotten to sell was a perquisite of leper hospitals in Scotland: wild beasts found dead or wounded, and rotten pork or salmon brought to market belonged by Act of Parliament to "ye hous of ye lepir men", if one existed in the district.

A corn levy, which in 1650 amounted to 546 tuns, was made on parishes surrounding Själö hospital in south-west Finland: parishes near the coast delivered their contributions by boat in the autumn; those further away inland waited until winter, because sledge was the easiest form of overland transport. Viborg leper hospital claimed four bushels of corn from each household in the county of Savonlinna, and about 50 farms belonging to or entailed to the hospital paid rent in corn, fish, butter, and wood. Various local windfalls contributed to the economy of leper hospitals, such as wreckage salvaged from a ship stranded on the Åland islands in 1657. Other occasional fruits of the sea included a whale on the Faroe islands each time a school was driven ashore and one eighth of each fisherman's catch on a nominated day in Iceland, provided the catch on that day was not less than five good-sized cod. In return for their obligations to the local hospital the parishes received the right to send their lepers there, a right illustrated by King Hans' decree concerning the lepers of Næstved in Denmark in 1492 (5), which stated that all lepers in parishes which paid rent to the hospital were to be admitted to it. As late as the early nineteenth century, parishes around Bergen in Norway still paid a regular tax in return for the right to send their lepers to St. George's hospital in Bergen.

Gifts of livestock, food, and money were welcome but rarely of great consequence. Bequests were common and provide the major source of knowledge of medieval leper hospitals. Henry II, who had the murder of Archbishop Becket on his conscience, left legacies to several hospitals, and his son William Longespee followed his example by bequeathing cattle to the leper hospitals at Salisbury, Maiden Bradley, and Wilton. The leper women of Maiden Bradley (it was one of the few institutions restricted to women) sponsored a weekly market and an annual fair from which they received tolls. Several other hospitals did likewise, notably the leper hospital of St. Mary Magdalene at Stourbridge near Cambridge, the church of which survives as Barnwell chapel, and whose name lives on in the annual Stourbridge fair.

It was usual for hospitals to own farms which were tended either by their healthy members, by paid servants, or were leased out. Few of the lepers would have been strong enough to work on the farm. Initially, the incomes of the hospitals were probably sufficient to pay for hired labour, but in the fourteenth century both the wealth of the hospitals and the availability of labour diminished; at the same time wages soared. Probably for these reasons "healthy brothers and sisters" were admitted in increasing numbers to do the work in return for food and lodging, as at Svendborg in Denmark where in 1486 there were eight healthy brothers and sisters "who shall nurse and work for their living". Many were probably relatives of the lepers, although these may sometimes have been admitted as a separate category; at Næstved in Denmark for example, separate reference is made to "the womenfolk" of the "sick brothers and sisters" and to the "healthy brothers and sisters". All capable inmates of Enköping hospital were expected to "help and work together with their own hands in summer and autumn to bring in the hay and to harvest the grain in wagons to the granary".

Many hospitals appointed a proctor to collect rents and to solicit alms; he was in effect the hospital's licensed beggar, an important privilege when begging was harshly controlled. In some areas the lepers themselves were also permitted by royal privilege to beg, particularly in the reign of King John, but this right was usually limited to the immediate vicinity of the hospital. As late as 1427, for example, a law of the Scottish parliament restricted begging by lepers to their own premises and to outlying districts; they were forbidden to beg in church, churchyard, or in the town. And at the end of the following century the lepers at Edinburgh were only permitted to beg at the gate of their hospital, a task which they undertook turn and turn about.

The proctor was usually chosen from the healthy members of a hospital community, but sometimes a leper was appointed, as at Beccles where a royal charter authorised one of the lepers to beg on behalf of his fellows. Generally it is not clear whether the proctor was a leper or not. At Berwick-on-Tweed, in the late thirteenth century, it is simply recorded that "some gude man" should gather alms on behalf of the lepers. A document dated April 23rd, 1384, under the common seal of the "Hospital of Leprous Persons of the blessed Mary Magdalene of Totnes", records the appointment by the master, brethren, and sisters of the hospital of "a proctor for conducting their causes and affairs". At Svendborg in Denmark the proctor was also elected by his companions; his function, as is strongly implied in the Totnes document also, was more administration than fund-raising, and it was the healthy brothers and sisters who were responsible for begging alms. English leper hospitals retained the right to appoint two proctors to gather alms until the privilege was abolished in 1597.

Thus over the years the office of proctor gradually evolved from itinerant alms-gatherer to resident administrator, often supplanting the warden who in many cases was no longer either resident or closely involved in the day-to-day affairs of the hospital. The "Pamphlet of the offices and duties of every particular sworn officer of the city of Exeter, collected by John Vowell, alias Hooker, Gent., chamberlain of the same", records that in 1584 the warden of the "Magdalene" (Plate 10) was appointed annually by the mayor and town council to govern and rule the hospital, either by "himself or his sufficient deputy". The master or warden of Sherburn hospital was often a man of such eminence and involvement in other spheres as certainly to have been non-resident, but in an institution so well staffed by clerics it really did not matter if the office of warden was a sinecure. One master, John de Waltham, resigned in 1384 to become bishop of Salisbury, a post which he could not have obtained simply by faithful service within Sherburn leper hospital. The most blatant sinecural appointment as master of Sherburn was that of Dr. Roderick Gundisalve, chargé d'affairs of the Spanish court. He was appointed by King Henry VII who, in the opinion of a historian of the hospital, "being a frugal prince, chose rather to reward foreigners who had been sent here on legations ... with preferments that cost nothing, than to impair his treasure by making pecuniary presents to them". Sherburn was, however, an exceptional institution in many respects, not least in regard to its affluence.

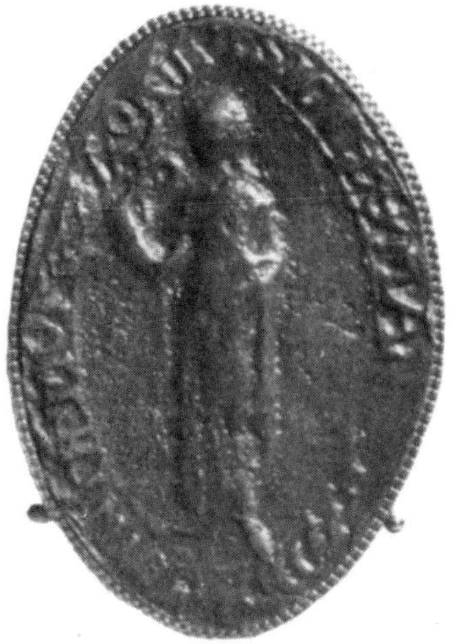

Plate 10a. Thirteenth-century seal of the hospital of St. Mary Magdalene, Exeter.

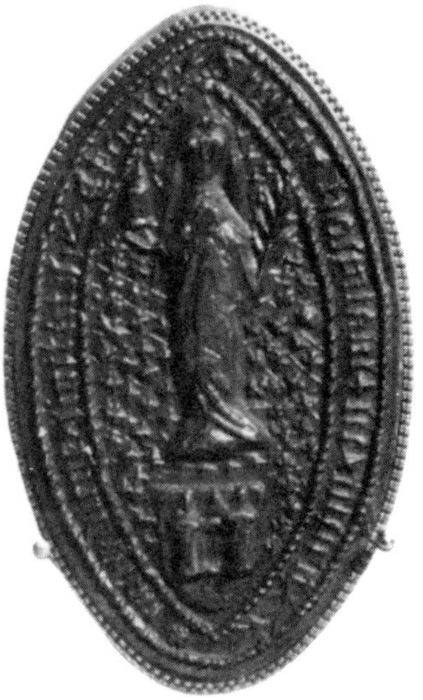

Plate 10b. Fifteenth-century seal of the hospital of St. Mary Magdalene, Exeter.

Towards the end of the Middle Ages the names and functions of proctor and pardoner became confused. The church had long swelled the revenues of leper hospitals by granting indulgences, either in return for cash payments to the hospital or for attendance at services in the hospital chapel, at which, naturally, almsgiving would be expected. Early documents refer to remittance of penance for seven or thirteen days; but inflation did not even spare indulgences and forty days remission became the standard. Pope Alexander IV later introduced an indulgence which was inflation-proof in a novel and important respect: benefactors of Allington leper hospital near Bridport in Dorset were offered a fractional remission of total penance instead of a fixed number of days, a considerable attraction to a man well-endowed both in sins and riches:

"Item, to all thos that gevyn broche, rynge, boke, belle, candell, vestimente, bordclothe, towelle, pygge, lambe, wolle, peny or penyworthe, be whiche the sayde hous and hospitale is amended and mentaynde, the sayd Pope grantethe the remission of the VII th parte of penance injunct". (6)

In due course hospital proctors became purveyors of indulgences, often, it seems, counterfeit. Those who purchased a pardon from the proctor of St. John's hospital, Canterbury (not itself a leper hospital) were credited with 30,000 paternosters and ave marias. Abuses multiplied to such an extent that in the mid-fourteenth century

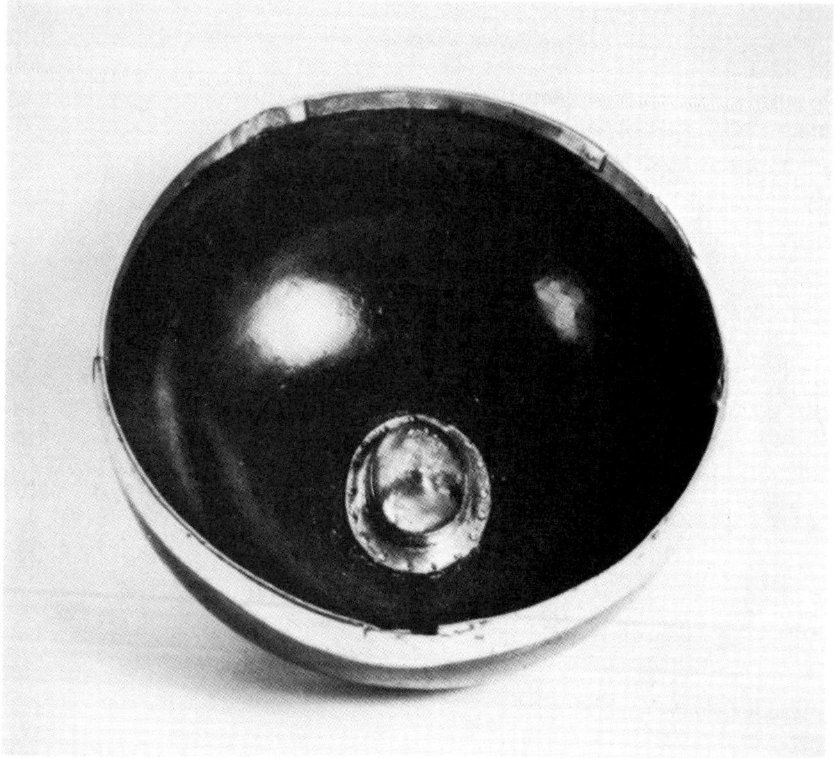

Plate 11. The Becket Shoe Mazer from St. Nicholas, Harbledown. This crystal, now set into a fourteenth-century mazer, was shown to Erasmus when he passed the hospital shortly before 1519.

Bishop Grandison of Exeter forbade those collecting alms in his diocese either to preach or to sell fictitious privileges and unauthorised pardons. Small wonder that both the people and their language became so confused about the offices of proctor and pardoner that in 1573 reference was made to a sum "paid to a pardoner that gathered for the hospital of Plympton".

A wide variety of tolls, taxes, and fines also benefited the hospitals. The lepers of St. Mary Magdalene at Southampton were due one penny for each tun of wine imported. A household tax called "leprosy money" was imposed on all households in the region of Åbo, and was said to be levied "in the same way as elsewhere". Scandinavian leper hospitals sometimes received legal fines, such as the fine or possessions of anyone executed at the local court which were given to St. George's hospital in Svendborg. In Finland two offenders, Clas Munk and Anders Hare, were ordered in 1623 to pay between them the very substantial sum of 500 daler to Själö hospital in mitigation of a crime. Free-will offerings were another source of ready-money. At Enköping hospital mazers were placed hopefully around the church and churchyard. Almsboxes were placed in the churches and harbours of Åland for the benefit of Gloskär leper hospital.

Some hospitals, such as Harbledown, were particularly well situated to gather alms from passing travellers. Harbledown hospital, the church of which still stands, was placed beside the London to Dover road just north of the city of Canterbury. Both pilgrims on their way to the shrine of Thomas Becket and travellers bound for France passed its gate. The first notable pilgrim (40 marks donated to the hospital) was King Henry II himself on his penitential pilgrimage to Canterbury. Early in the sixteenth century Erasmus of Rotterdam visited Canterbury. As he passed Harbledown hospital one of the brethren ran out, sprinkled him with holy water and proffered a disintegrating shoe in which was set "a piece of glass resembling a jewel". Erasmus was invited to kiss the shoe, which was claimed to be the shoe of St. Thomas, the martyr (7). What better inducement to charity than this relic? Whether Becket's shoe-buckle ornament or not, this crystal has survived set into a fourteenth-century maplewood mazer (Plate 11).

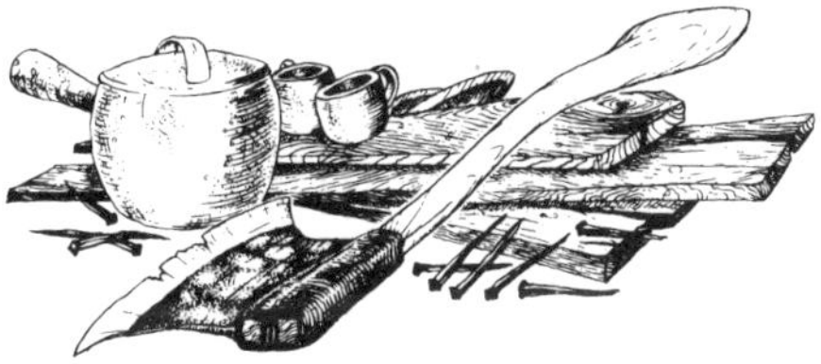

V

Sentence and Certificates

No tradition bound seventeenth-century Åland more firmly to the Middle Ages than the convention that the stringency of isolation should be determined by the certainty of diagnosis. Medieval medical textbooks, of which Guy de Chauliac's work (1) published in 1363 was the most influential, laid down two principles. First, anyone found on examination to have been wrongly accused of leprosy was to receive a certificate of freedom from the disease. Second, findings of doubtful significance merited observation at home; stronger suspicion was sufficient for the sentence *cassatus* to be pronounced, and for the suspect to be strictly isolated at home; finally, when no doubt remained, the leper must "with kind and consoling words" be sent to hospital. It is not clear why sentence was pronounced before the diagnosis was confirmed, nor is it apparent at what stage of certainty the church insisted on the ritual seclusion of the leper. Medical textbooks assumed that doctors would make the diagnosis, an assumption which ignored the fact that only large towns had qualified doctors, and that their services would be too expensive for most suspects. In the country, particularly in isolated districts, the people had no alternative but to decide the matter for themselves.

Even in the relatively rare situation when an expert medical opinion was obtained, importance was also attached to lay opinion. Early in the fourteenth century Peter de Nutle, lately mayor of Winchester, was accused by his successor and the city bailiffs of being a leper. He satisfied his accusers that he did not have the disease by submitting to examination by both lay and medical assessors. An order for his redress served on the civic authorities states that "from the inspection and examination before our council by the council and by physicians expert in the knowledge of this disease, the said Peter is whole and clean, and infected in no part of his body". Consequently the sheriff of Hampshire was directed to proclaim Peter de Nutle's innocence, so that he might live in peace where he wished. A royal mandate of 1346 stipulated that "men of knowledge" should inquire into suspected cases, but it should not be presumed that medical experience is implied, other than that acquired by any competent grandmother. In fact the later case of Joanna Nightingale indicates that assessment by laymen was the rule.

In 1468, Joanna Nightingale of Brentwood in Essex was accused by her neighbours of being "infected by the foul contact of leprosy". Joanna, clearly a woman of spirit, refused either to be inspected or to withdraw from the community. Her neighbours petitioned for her removal by a writ of *De leproso amovendo*, and a Chancery warrant was issued in the name of King Edward IV for her "to be diligently viewed and examined" in the presence of "certain discreet and loyal men of the county"; no suggestion was made that these should be medical men. At this point the Lord Chancellor himself intervened in the case. His intervention is probably an indication of the rarity of such a case at that time rather than a sign of Joanna's importance. The inexpert approach to diagnosis may particularly have alarmed his Lordship, for he arranged that the royal physicians should examine Joanna.

Medicine had advanced so little that the physicians assessed her condition strictly according to the time-worn criteria of de Chauliac. Indeed, the philosophy of medical diagnosis progressed little between 1350 and 1850, let alone between the publication of de Chauliac's work in 1363 and the case of Joanna Nightingale in 1468; medievalism maintained a firm grip on both men's minds and their medicine long after the Middle Ages. But such has been the recent revolution of medical science that there is now hardly a disease which could be approached adequately by the criteria of one hundred years ago.

After carefully weighing all the symptoms and signs the royal physicians concluded that Joanna neither was nor had been a leper and therefore should not be separated from the community. Thus William Hatticlyff, Roger Marshall and Dominus de Serego signed their names and set their seals on the earliest English medical certificate to survive (2).

The writ issued against Joanna Nightingale in the closing years of the Middle Ages reveals the normal procedure for accusing and assessing lepers. Neighbours accused, and responsible and worthy citizens examined. In Scotland in the late sixteenth and early seventeenth centuries two different practices existed. In some places, as in Glasgow, the magistrates were responsible for searching for, assessing, and consigning lepers to hospital: they ordered in 1573 that people suspected to have leprosy were "to be viseit and gif they be found so, to be secludit of the town to the hospital at the Brigend". Further north, as in Aberdeen, the parish meeting assumed this mantle: for example on May 13th, 1604, the Kirk session ordered "Helene Smythe, ane puir woman infectit with Leprosie to be put in the hospital appoyntit for keeping and handling lipper folkis betwixt the townis".

Priest and people were the normal judge and jury of leprosy in most parts of Scotland and Scandinavia in the seventeenth and eighteenth centuries, a custom which continued the usual medieval practice; doctors were rarely involved. Bishops, deans, and other ecclesiastical officers were required by the act of the Scottish Parliament *Anent Lipper Folke* to "inquyre diligentlie" on their visits to the parishes whether anyone was "smitted with lipper". In remote communities, such as on the Shetland isles, the Kirk sessions took upon themselves the legal powers conferred upon the higher clergy. The session of the parish of Walls on December 6th, 1772, recorded that

> "This day the session being informed that Margaret Abernethy, relick spouse of James Henry, had been to all appearance for a considerable time past, deeply tinted with the inveterate scurvy, commonly called the Leprosy in this place, and was now removed to Brabaster in the midst of a number of children, whose parents were in the greatest fear of their being infected with the disease by the said Margaret Abernethy. And that they and others had again called on the session to convene the said woman before them in order to be sighted, and also to be set apart if she be found unclean, to conform to the former use and wont in this and other parishes of the country. Therefore the session did and hereby do appoint the officer to require the said Margaret Abernethy to compear before

them at this place next Wednesday in order to be examined and inspected as above said." (3)

In short, the parishioners accused, and the parish council both examined and passed sentence, but now only when doubt remained.

The lines of Pastor Muur's diary of his parish visitations echo both those "discrete and loyal men" chosen to examine Joanna Nightingale and the members of the Kirk session on Shetland, for on Åland too the parishioners themselves were the judge and jury of leprosy in the community. On the few occasions when a suspect was unable or unwilling to attend a general meeting of the parish for questioning and inspection, men (never women apparently) of the parish were chosen to visit and inspect. For example, it was reported to the visiting dean and parish meeting at Föglö on February 29th, 1640, that "Housewife Kaarin who was suspected to be a leper sleeps in the same room as others in the house. It is reported that she refuses to be separated from them. Herr Erich, Herr Gabriel, and several other good men are instructed to travel there to acquaint her with the regulations and to report as soon as possible that they have done so." The proposed examination of Joanna at Brentwood in 1468, the action of the parish meeting at Walls in Shetland in 1772, and this meeting of the parish of Föglö on Åland in 1640, all bear striking witness to a common medieval tradition. Kaarin was not an exceptional case. Sund parish meeting in 1650 decided that "Cnut's wife in Finby" who had been under observation for three years "should be examined by men appointed by the sheriff's officer". Again at Sund, on March 18th, 1655, an order was given for Lisbeeta, also of Finby, to be inspected by the sheriff's officer and some good men as soon as possible.

Suspicion of a parishioner was aroused either by evasive behaviour or by rumour, and once rumours were circulating they doubtless, like the one feather of Hans Andersen's story, rapidly grew into five hens. Märtha of Önningeby was suspected to have leprosy in 1640 because she had not been seen in church for two years; the parish may have had good reason for suspecting leprosy rather than dissent as the cause of her absence. At Sund on February 3rd, 1660, Muur was told that "People have been spreading rumours about Anna of Månstekta, and they fight shy of her in the church pew. She has been told to leave the pew and to stand by herself at the back of the church". Poor ostracised Anna, she was sufficiently suspect to have her company shunned, but not so tainted that the parish was prepared to lose a good pair of hands: Muur recorded that "in spite of this she has promised to take part in the farm work until God's work can be seen". Formal sentence (they used the same word as de Chauliac, with all its legal force) was never passed on Anna; she died after four years of observation, but whether of leprosy or of some other disease will never be known. Kirsten of Söderby is named as a suspect at the parish meeting of Lemland on May 18th, 1653, with the curt note that she "is being avoided by others". Her diagnosis was soon confirmed, and she was sentenced a leper the next year, eventually dying in the hospital at Gloskär on March 3rd, 1660.

Once suspicion had been aroused, investigation and formal assessment were in the hands of the parish meeting. When a formal sentence of leprosy had been passed the church authorities were informed, and they in turn notified the civic authorities. Muur revealed the procedure when on February 7th, 1650, he wrote—

> "Today I record that the sheriff has sent me to make this inspection visit which I am holding today at Lemland, armed with a copy of His Majesty's strict order 'Concerning lepers'. Each parish must give their verdict annually without fail, so that they never need to wait for the priest. Immediately afterwards a report should be sent to the priest together with notification of the day he was sentenced and whether his means amount to the 50 daler required for his keep." (4)

The parish priest himself was rarely mentioned as party to the verdict-making, probably because he was *ex officio* a member of the parish meeting, and did not therefore need special mention. Only once, on May 18th, 1653, were "the priest and parish council" together instructed to call a parishioner for examination. The "priest" who was to be formally notified of the verdict of the parish was the rural dean, and his further duties in the matter were as follows:

> "It is the priest's duty to make a note of the sentence and its date, and to notify the sheriff who will then give instructions concerning subsistence and removal under the supervision of the priest. When they have been removed the priest shall certify the fact with his signature. If any parish or person tries to hinder the execution of these regulations, then each must answer for his disobedience." (4)

The parish priest was responsible for ensuring that isolation at home was effective. At Hammarland on March 25th, 1640, Muur recorded that "A leprous housewife in Stromma is confined to bed and lives with her husband. Her husband travels all over the district and is not at present in the parish. The parish priest was instructed to enforce the order against them": either the woman had been ordered to live apart from her husband, or her husband had been instructed not to travel away from home—in any event it was the rector who was expected to deal with the matter. On the other hand, lepers who moved from parish to parish were the responsibility of the civil authorities. In 1657, for example, the sheriff was asked by the parish of Lemland to stop lepers travelling about without permission.

The parish normally called a general meeting outside the church for the formal examination of a suspected leper. It must have been an awesome event. In the presence of Muur, who was visiting Önningeby, the parish meeting on March 22nd, 1640, sent instructions that Märtha must present herself on the mound by the church to give an account of herself, so that "she could be either cleared or sentenced". As far as can be judged from Muur's notes the examination was partly a superficial medical examination with interrogation and scrutiny of visible parts, and partly an investigation of financial circumstances. Sunday was the usual day: an examination for leprosy doubtless added a little spice to an otherwise routine visit to church. In 1648, a woman called Kaisa was ordered by the parish of Föglö to "present herself by the church wall on the next Sunday so that the people can decide whether she is leprous or whether she should remain under observation": there seemed to be no question of a reprieve in her case, perhaps having been under observation in her home for three years already they felt instinctively that it was only a question of time before convincing proof was obtained. Both on that occasion, and evidently the next year too, their verdict was simply that home isolation should be continued. Thus passed her fourth and fifth years as an outcast. Not until 1650 did Muur, on another visit to Föglö, sound the more hopeful note that Kaisa was again "going to be inspected on Sunday and either be freed or confirmed". Maybe her slender hope of freedom after five years waiting was fulfilled because Kaisa is never heard of again, and her name does not appear in the list of those admitted either to Gloskär or Själö hospitals. Not every inspection took place on a Sunday: at Jomala in 1653, Karin of Svilby was "ordered to submit herself to inspection on Ascension Day and to accept the verdict of the parish".

Sentence was formal and momentous; it signified such certainty of leprosy that an order was made forthwith for removal to hospital, as in the case of "Erich Anderson of Storby and Maria Tomazdotter of Maarby", who in 1655 were sentenced "in front of a good many parishioners ... and must be taken away". On one remarkable occasion, at Sund in 1649, Hinder Hindersson of Finby, was sentenced at least partly on his own testimony, for he openly admitted that he was a leper. Up and down the islands, year by year, new suspects were assessed, and others already under observation were reviewed "according to the judgement of the parish". Usually their names were recorded and sometimes their occupations too, such as the widow, the soldier's daughter, and the boatman summoned to appear before the parish meeting at Ekerö in 1649.

Those who could afford the journey obtained permission to sail to Stockholm for medical examination. In matters of medical authority Åland still looked to Stockholm. Several made the journey in an attempt to avoid indecisive years of home isolation. Some, doubtless vainly, hoped to persuade themselves and others that they did not have the disease which they recognised but could not accept. From all these voyages only one record exists of a certificate of freedom successfully procured and accepted by the parish as proof of good health. At a meeting of the parish of Hammarland on February 3rd, 1657, Muur wrote that "Anders Henriksson of Posta has been declared by the parish to be free of the leprosy of which he had been accused on the grounds of the certificate he procured in Stockholm". Others in the parish were encouraged by his success, for the next year when Muur passed through he learnt that Bertil Skinnare, one of those under home observation, was in Stockholm for examination and two girls had been given leave to travel there for the same purpose. The parents of a boy suspected of leprosy were currently deliberating whether to send him to Stockholm, or whether to submit without argument to the demand of the parish that he should be sent to stay with another person already under observation. And what if the poor boy did not have leprosy and the other suspect did?

As time went on the parishes seemed to encourage suspects to seek proper medical assessment in Stockholm. One can imagine the many excuses they made to their fellow passengers on the crowded ship in order to conceal the true purpose of their journey. The parish of Jomala was so insistent on proper medical diagnosis by 1664 that it declared "If the family will not take the boy in Lorningsöö, who is under observation on suspicion of leprosy, to Stockholm to be examined by a doctor, then they must be summoned to the district meeting and the assistance of the authorities should be sought in this matter." At Sund, on January 24th, 1664, two other suspects raised no objections: "Jacob of Gesterby and Matz Hinderson of Finby have both been placed under observation by the parish meeting with their own consent and agreement. On the first day of spring they will both travel to Stockholm to be examined by an experienced doctor." The first day of spring doubtless came when the ice melted. Neither of these men appear in the records of Gloskär; Matz Hinderson probably stayed at Stockholm for treatment and never returned, for the disease was in the family; Margretha Matzdotter from the same village of Finby, who three years later was sentenced a leper and sent to Gloskär, was almost certainly his daughter.

Medical examination had been customary for confirmation of a diagnosis of leprosy in Stockholm since at least 1482, when the civic authorities instructed a barber-surgeon to inspect Henrik Mulle and several others. Mulle's diagnosis was confirmed and he was admitted to St. George's hospital. In acknowledgement of his fate he bequeathed all his worldly possessions to his son-in-law four days later. But where resources are scarce, progress must wait; no medical examination of a leper on the Åland islands is recorded in the seventeenth century.

In Finland itself during the seventeenth century medical confirmation of the diagnosis gradually became the normal procedure. Bishop Gezelius decreed in 1673 that suspects should not be released from isolation until they had been cleared by the "doctor and surgeon". In 1675, three years after the Åland lepers had been transferred from Gloskär to Själö hospital in south-west Finland, Elias Tillandz, professor of medicine at Åbo university, was sent on behalf of the Crown to examine these new arrivals. The reason for this high-level examination was not to exclude possible injustice through inexpert diagnosis on Åland, but to see whether any might be discharged to save the Crown the cost of supporting them; it is a tribute to the accuracy of diagnosis by the people of Åland that no discharges are recorded. Tillandz visited again in 1686, and in 1704 his successor, Prof. N. Wallerius, who was considered a specialist in leprosy, visited the hospital. In 1725, Bishop Witte of Åbo was accompanied on his inspection visit to Själö hospital by both the professor of medicine, P. Elfving, and by the provincial surgeon, H. L. Geitel.

Not only were lepers in hospital now sporadically examined medically but parishes in south-west Finland sent their suspects to the professor of medicine at Åbo for his decision, such as a 15-year-old boy from Kimito who was sent to Prof. Hielm in 1706. Another certificate signed in 1734 by Prof. H. D. Spöring of Åbo, author of the first medical case-report of leprosy in Scandinavia (see p. 100), confirms that "Beata Hans dotter has leprosy and should therefore withdraw from the company of others" (5). Other towns which possessed neither university nor professor made do with a more pragmatic (and perhaps no less effective) diagnostician; in Viborg for example, an inmate of the hospital was moved from the "clean" side to the leprous after examination by the city's barber surgeon.

Memories of the disease were still green in England in the seventeenth century, although leprosy itself was probably dead. No local physician or barber surgeon remained competent to diagnose the disease, and it was to doctors in London that people now looked for an authoritative opinion. How often suspects travelled there for examination is not known, but the chance survival of one long-forgotten certificate introduces one such plaintiff, and it is unlikely that he was unique. This certificate, given in 1620 to Nicholas Harris, footpostman of Totnes, was briefly cited in a paper given to the Devonshire Association in 1880 (6). It was clearly a document of the greatest interest, but a search in 1972 revealed no trace of it.

In March 1974, when almost all hope of finding it had been abandoned, Nicholas Harris' certificate (7) was rediscovered in a sheaf of Victorian documents amongst Totnes papers in the Devon Record Office. It was in the form of a petition (Plate 12) presented to the Royal College of Physicians of London. Harris was either very uncertain as to which "good testymony" would adequately "certifie that I

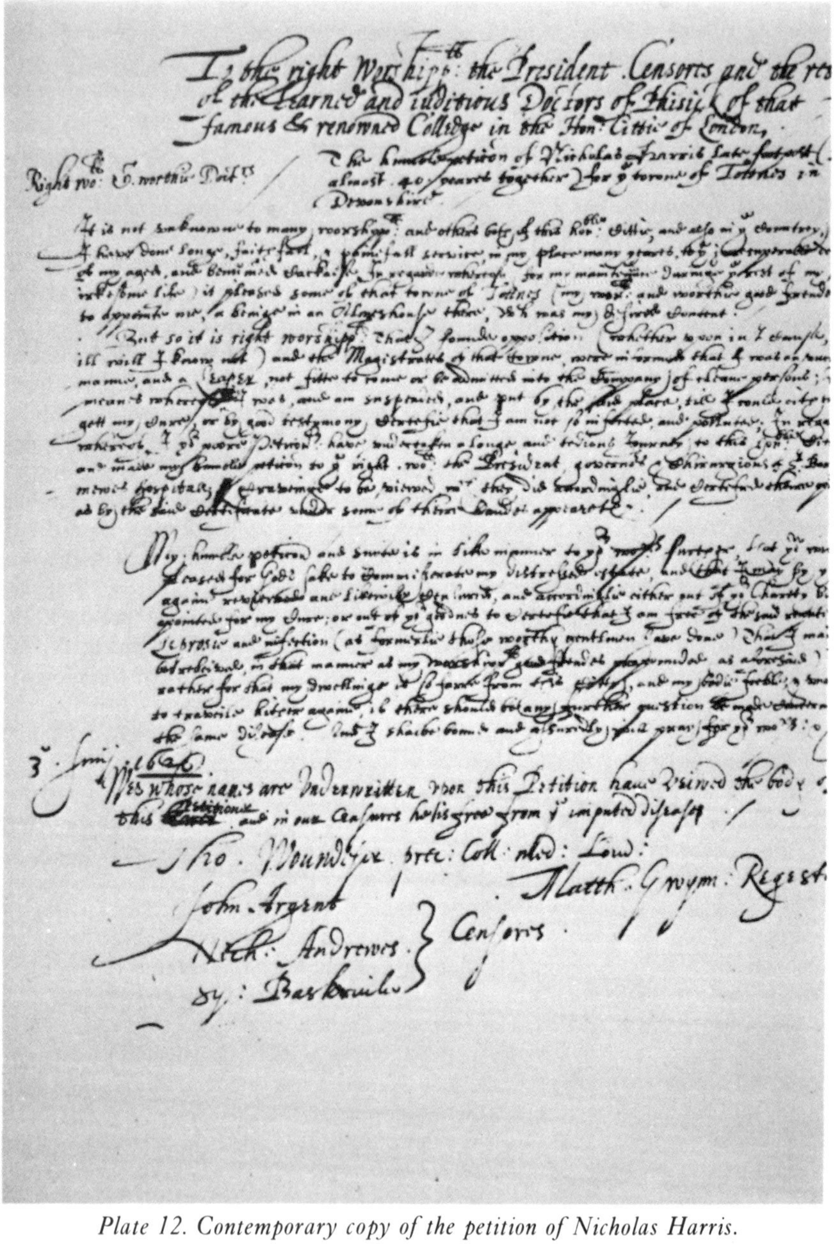
To the right Worshipp^ll the President, Censors and the rest of the learned and judicious Doctors of Phisick of that famous & renowned Colledge in the Hon. Cittie of London,

Tho. Moundford Pres: Coll: Med: Lond:
John Argent
Rich: Andrewes
Censors
Matth. Gwynn Regist

Plate 12. Contemporary copy of the petition of Nicholas Harris.

am not so infected and polluted", or determined to ensure that his absolution was secured both by belt and braces. His caution was indeed reasonable, for the 193 miles from Totnes to London was a "long and tedious journey" to be sure, especially considering that he had relinquished his duties as footpost on account of the "irresuperable decay" of his "aged and binumed carkaise". Harris was keenly aware that his "bodie feeble" could never undertake such a journey again if further doubts should be raised about his health on his return home.

He first found his way to St. Bartholomew's hospital, where he was examined by "ye right worshippfull the President, governors and chirurgions", and obtained their certificate that he was not a leper. He then composed (or more likely dictated to a notary) a petition to be viewed by the "President, Censores and the rest of the learned and juditious Doctors of Phisick of that famous and renowned Colledge in the Hon: Cittie of London"—in short, the Royal College of Physicians. Perhaps someone had whispered that the governors and surgeons of St. Bartholomew's were no longer the highest authorities on medical diagnosis in the land.

The most affluent and celebrated doctor could not have resisted his humble and touching petition. He explained that on completing his "longe, faitefull and painfull service" as footpost for nearly forty years he had been recommended for a place in a Totnes almshouse. But, "whether upon just cause or ill will I know not", someone had informed the local magistrate that he was "an uncleane manne and a Leaper, not fitte to come or be admitted into the company of cleane persons". Thus consideration of his application was deferred until he obtained either a cure or a certificate that he was free from the disease.

On June 3rd, 1620, his petition was endorsed by Thomas Moundeford, President of the Royal College of Physicians, Matthew Gwynn, Registrar, and John Argent, Richard Andrewes and Sidney Baskerville, Censors, with these words: "Wee whose names are underwritten upon this Petition have viewed the body of this petitioner and in our censurrs he is free from ye imputed diseases." With lighter heart Nicholas Harris retraced his steps to Totnes. Cautious to the last, he presented to the authorities not the certificate itself but the copy which has survived three hundred and fifty years longer than Nicholas himself. He ended his days peacefully in the almshouse—"which was my desired content".

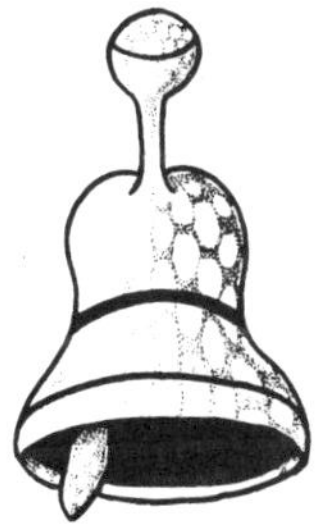

VI

Separation

The convention that lepers should be separated from society runs through eight centuries of European history. There the superficial unity ends; the reasons for separation have differed, not only with the passing of time, but even in neighbouring countries at the same time. Thus, any one place at any one period gives only part of a complicated picture, and to generalise from it can be very misleading. The tradition that fear of infection was the common key to the isolation of lepers is an over-simplification. No aspect of the leper's history is more important, because attitudes towards him were closely bound up with the reasons for setting him apart.

By the seventeenth century, fear of infection had indeed become the prime reason for separation. Thus in this respect the Åland islands, where fear was unmistakable, were not typical of the Middle Ages. The motive for separation in the early Middle Ages was essentially religious, founded on the linguistic and ritualistic confusions discussed earlier, and formalised in Levitical law (Plate 13). Åland,

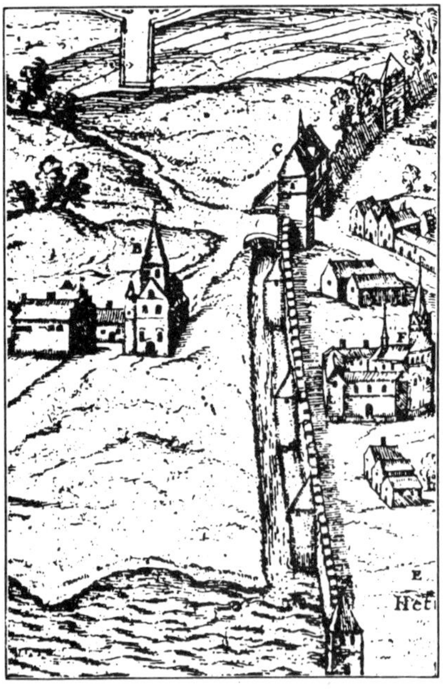

Plate 13. St. George's hospital, Visby, Sweden, about 1600, showing its situation outside the city wall.

true to its rôle as a channel of medieval thought and practice into later centuries, still remembered this principle, although it was no longer the driving force of the people's actions. On March 1st, 1640, several "good men" of Föglö parish were sent to inspect a woman suspected of leprosy who refused to live apart from her family. They returned the following day and reported to the parish that she had promised to live in isolation in her own house "according to the Levitical law"—and they quoted chapter and verse. Only when her diagnosis was finally confirmed and she was sentenced a leper would the secular law committing all lepers to hospital apply to her, a law founded by that time upon fear of infection, not upon religious law.

The Church had reinforced the Levitical law in a decree of the Lateran Council under Pope Alexander III in 1179 (confirmed at Westminster in 1200), instructing that a leper should not mix with others, share their church, or be buried with them. A leper was not initially bound to enter hospital, but he was required to cut himself off from society. As very few lepers could afford home isolation most were forced to seek shelter and support in an institution.

Priests who caught leprosy, as some did, were more fortunate than other men because the Church provided for them. In this matter, as in all others, priests were subject only to ecclesiastical law. The bishop together with a "coadjudicator" of his own choosing was responsible for deciding the fate of clergy accused of the disease in his diocese. A Swedish archbishop, Andreas Suneson of Lund, once retired to self-imposed isolation on suspicion of leprosy. According to Icelandic tradition, two early bishops of Skalkholt in Iceland became lepers, not as unlikely an event as it may sound because five hundred years later Jón Petersen, an Icelandic blacksmith's son, reported as a medical student that three parish priests in his homeland had developed leprosy within a period of eight years: one died in 1764, another four years later, and the third had recently written to him describing his symptoms. Leprosy in priests was not necessarily an occupational disease; Petersen noted that one of them had a leprous mother.

Iceland experienced in the eighteenth century what England had not seen since the Middle Ages. Several English parish priests had been suspended from their duties because they had leprosy, and a bishop would certainly not lightly confirm the diagnosis in an incumbent. But once the disease had assumed its characteristic features the parishioners were as good a judge as any man, and their complaint had to be investigated. Priests were suspended because of leprosy at Seyton in the diocese of Lincoln in 1310, St. Neot and Colyton in the diocese of Exeter in 1314 and 1330 respectively, and at Castle Carrock in Carlisle in 1357. Pope Clement III had ordered that parish priests removed from their livings on account of leprosy should be maintained out of the income of their benefices, a potentially heavy burden on the leper-priest's successor for this was characteristically a prolonged disease. Sir Philip, the rector of St. Neot suspended in 1314, was allowed two shillings per week together with twenty shillings annually for clothing. Besides this pecuniary allowance he retained the best room in the vicarage; the house was divided and the curate lived in the other part with no communication between them. In Norway in 1339, Bishop Håkon of Bergen removed a leprous priest from his living; he undertook to provide for him and permitted him to live wherever he wished.

Ecclesiastical and common law agreed that lepers should be separated from the community. But the disease only became an offence under English common law (and the same was true in medieval Scandinavia) if a leper insisted on dwelling in a town, attending church, or mixing with his neighbours. In those circumstances lepers could be removed by force under a writ of *De leproso amovendo*, provided that by their disfigurement they "appear to the sight of all men that they are lepers". Heretics, a less common nuisance, could be burned under a writ of *De haeretico comburendo* (abolished as late as 1677), but the leper could only be cast out.

A few records of proceedings against individuals under a writ of *De leproso amovendo* have survived. One of the earliest was the action at the Curia Regis in 1220 in which William, son of Nicholas Malesmains, was committed to the hospital of St. Mary Magdalene at Bidelington. Others, such as Richard, Alice and Matilda, who wished in spite of their disease to remain in the town "to the great damage and prejudice of the inhabitants", were expelled from Gloucester in 1273, and Thomas Tytel Webstere of Norwich was expelled in 1375. The Assizes of London declared in 1276 that "no leper shall be in the city, nor come there, nor make any stay there", a bye-law which was confirmed by Edward III in 1346, who proclaimed that anyone proved leprous must leave within 15 days, whatever their station in life, "and betake themselves to places in the country, solitary and notably distant from the city and suburbs".

Bye-laws forbidding lepers to live within the town were common, such as those recorded in the "Customs of Bristol" in 1344. Scottish local laws were similar and quite as old. The twelfth century "Burrow Laws" required that "if any man dwelled or borne in the King's Burgh is stricken with leprosie ... he shall be put in the hospitall of that burgh where he dwells ... no man should be so bauld as to harberie or ludge ane lipperman within the burgh". The Canons of the Church of Scotland (1242-69) agreed that lepers should be "separated from society in accordance with general custom and retired to secluded situations". General custom may indeed have been far older than the papal pronouncement of 1179.

Although local bye-laws were generally similar they were by no means uniform, particularly in the early Middle Ages. In Exeter, for example, restriction of lepers was a matter for the bishop who, until 1244, allowed lepers free access to the town. He then acquiesced to pressure from the city council to transfer lepers to its jurisdiction. Permissive legislation was the exception, and the tolerance of the bishop of Exeter was only matched by two Scottish regulations. A canon of the thirteenth century indicated that if lepers were able to fulfil their parochial obligations then they should do so, but "if they cannot be induced to do so, let no coercion be employed, seeing that affliction should not be accumulated upon the afflicted, but rather their misfortunes commiserated". An act of the Perth parliament in Scotland is said to have given lepers the right to enter the town from 10 to 12 o'clock on Mondays, Wednesdays and Fridays.

After the standard church service which formally separated the leper (1), and before leading him to his place of isolation, the priest was required to read to the leper the rules governing his new existence in a world within yet outside the world he knew before. He was forbidden the company of others in church, market, mill, bakehouse, or tavern. If he wished to buy he must touch the article with his stick and receive it into his bowl; nothing and nobody must he touch with his bare hand. His dress and warning rattle (Plate 14) or bell (Plate 15) must declare him to be a leper and his feet must always be shod. If he stopped to talk to someone on the road he must stand to the leeward, and he must avoid narrow

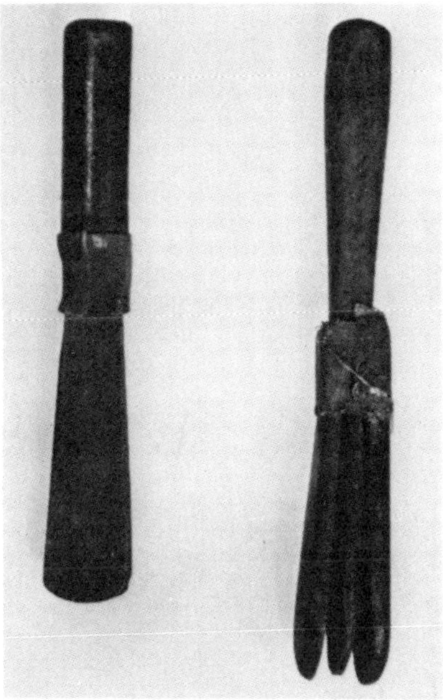

Plate 14. An English leper's clapper: facsimile of an original which used to be in the possession of the hospital at St. Nicholas, Harbledown.

lanes which might bring him into close contact with others. Apart from the companionship of his wife, the only company he now may keep in life, or in death, was that of other lepers.

These rules show that wherever a leper lived he was not strictly under house-arrest. Rules of many institutions confirm that those admitted to hospital in the early Middle Ages were not completely confined to the hospital precincts. A curious ambivalence of separation and participation pervades the regulations and warns against conclusions which seem self-evident today, but which may not have been logical to those concerned. At St. Julian's near St. Albans, for example, the leper brothers were forbidden to loiter on the path outside the hospital or to converse with others there, yet one at least of their number was permitted to visit the mill and brewery, another supervised the farm work, for which outside labourers were hired,.and all were entitled to seek leave from the master to visit St. Albans and even to spend a night away from the hospital.

Was it social or religious defilement, or was it fear of infection which determined the form of these limitations of the leper's freedom; or was it a subtle mixture of all three? Creighton, who did not himself believe that leprosy was an infectious disease, accepted that lepers were ostracised by public opinion and legislated against, but he warned that "The reality of these practices should not be confounded with a real need for them. Least of all should they be ascribed to a general belief in the contagiousness of the disease. In practice", he maintained, "no one heeded the medical dogma of leprous contagion because no one attached any concrete meaning to it or had any real experience of it." (2) Now his insistence that the reality of measures taken should not be confused with a real need for them is unimpeachable, but his view that because no one had a concrete understanding of the concept of infection, therefore no such concept popularly existed is unacceptable. Neither doctors nor medical dogma are needed to teach grandmothers

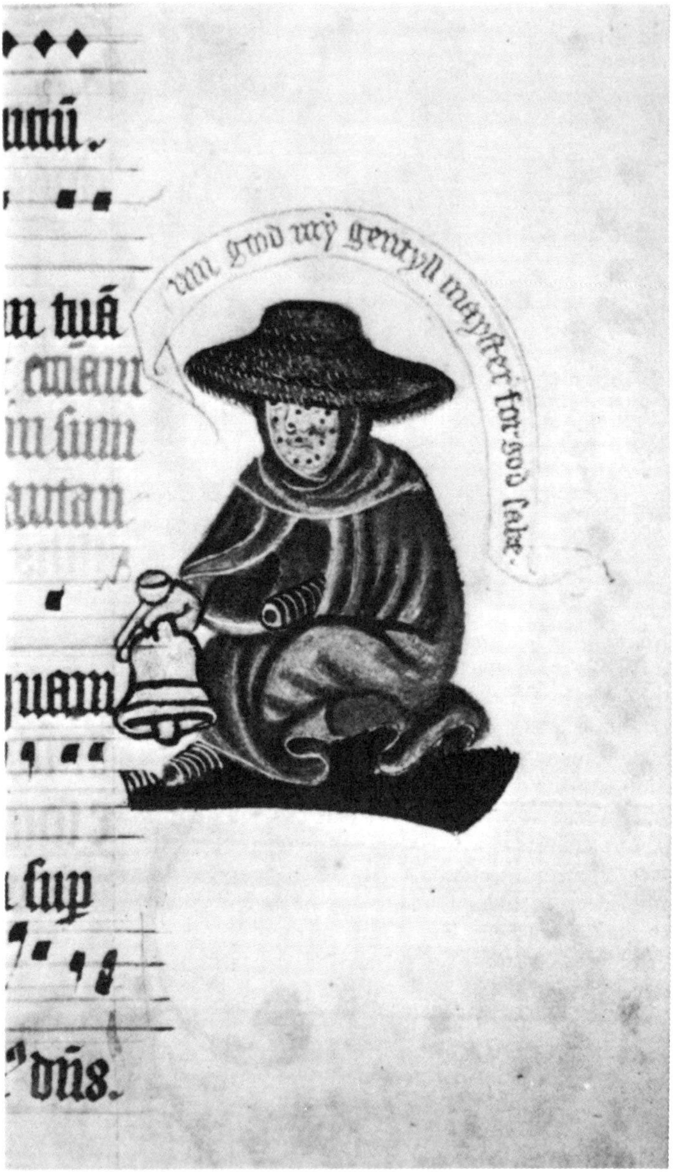

Plate 15. A leper with bell: marginal sketch in a fourteenth-century manuscript of the Exeter Pontifical.

about everyday diseases: did people really doubt that many childhood diseases spread from one child to another? And when the Black Death ravaged northern Europe was it doubted that it spread from person to person, regardless of the fact that both the causative bacteria and its different modes of transmission were unknown? Did a lack of concrete theory concerning the cause of leprosy release men and women from the instinctive fear that the horrible disfigurement which they saw in others might also take root in them?

Certainly, by the mid-fourteenth century, danger of infection was officially acknowledged: a mandate of Edward III in 1346 refers to contagion by polluted breath and by carnal intercourse, "to the great injury of the people ... and the manifest peril of other persons" (3), but just how great the danger seemed to the man in the street is not certain. He may have been no more concerned about the risk of acquiring leprosy than the citizens of York had been in the dangers inherent in the "abominable smell abounding in the said city more than in any other city in the realm from dung and manure and other filth and dirt wherewith the streets and lanes are filled and obstructed", which, in the opinion of Edward III in 1332, constituted a threat to "the health of the inhabitants and of those coming to the present parliament" (4).

Regardless of how much or little the people feared catching the disease, the church, the author of the standard rules, was primarily if not entirely concerned with religious implications. Nothing in the rules needs to be explained on any other grounds than the avoidance of defilement by an outcast, a concept unfamiliar today but very real then. The company of men, water, pathways, goods for sale, posts and gates, the air itself must not be polluted; even the burial place of the dead must not be defiled.

Early in the Middle Ages admission to hospital was considered something of a luxury, as the regulations of St. Julian's show by giving an order of preference for admission when a vacancy occurred. If a brother regarded the privilege of belonging to the house so lightly as to be absent without leave for twenty four hours, he could only be readmitted by the special permission of the abbot of St. Albans. Both at St. Julian's and at Sherburn hospital near Durham the ultimate punishment for disobedience was expulsion. Only once is the expulsion of a leper from hospital documented, and the fact that it was such a ceremonious occasion suggests that it was a rare event. The date of this ceremony at Ilford in Essex is not recorded, but an eighteenth century version of a contemporary account has survived. An impressive collection of ecclesiastical dignitaries was assembled to witness the just punishment of a leper caught with "a drab in his chamber".

> "The abbesse being accompanyed with the bishop of London, the abbot of Stratford, the deane of Paule's and other great spyrytuall personnes went to Ilford to visit the hospytall theere, founded for leepers; and uppon occacion of one of the lepers, who was a brother of the house, having brought into his chamber a drab, and sayd that she was his sister ... He came attyred in his lyvery, but bare-footed and bare-headed ... and was set on his knees uppon the stayres benethe the altar, where he remained during all the time of mass. When mass was ended, the prieste disgraded him of orders, scraped his hands and his crown with a knife, took his booke from him, gave him a boxe on the chiek with the end of his fingers, and then thrust him out of the churche, where the officers and people receyved him, and putt him into a carte, crying 'Ha rou, Ha rou, Ha rou', after him." (5)

Expulsion from hospital as a punishment denies any notion that the hospitals were founded to prevent the spread of infection. The detailed regulations of early medieval leper hospitals were primarily concerned with improving souls and caring for those who could not support themselves, not with containing infection. Most medieval hospitals whether for lepers or not, were religious foundations with similar regulations. Conformity was the keynote and some institutions demanded a formal vow, such as the vow of obedience ("unless any others are contrary to God's will") made by entrants to St. Julian's hospital to the abbot of St. Albans. Matters of misbehaviour considered worthy of individual mention in the St. Julian's regulations were theft, bearing false witness, violence, unchastity, alteration of bequests, renunciation of the abbot's absolute authority, and failure to keep bounds. Further, and perhaps unwisely, the entrant promised "to be satisfied without complaint or murmur with the food and drink and other things given me by the master".

In no aspect of daily life were the lepers more obviously part of a religious community than in their devotional obligations. These varied in detail from place to place but were heroic by modern standards—if not by monastic criteria. The regulations of Enköping hospital clearly stated the lepers' obligations:

> "... despising worldly things and dedicating themselves and their possessions to Christ they must ardently and freely devote themselves to vigils, fasting, prayers and other services, and to the promises of God." (6)

At Sherburn hospital, besides mass on holy days and feast days, the basic prescription of paternosters was 26 for matins, 14 for prime, 14 for nones, 18 for vespers and 14 for compline, together with 25 for their own sins and as many again for the souls of the bishops of Durham and for the faithful departed, a total of 161 daily. This was not all: on the death of a brother or sister a further 300 paternosters were to be said on his behalf over the next thirty days, an identical requirement to that at Svendborg in Denmark, where, however, the normal daily requirement was only about one third of the Sherburn duty. Dover leper hospital seems to have been the most demanding of all, requiring 200 paternosters and ave marias by day and as many again by night. Allowance was made for those whose ill-health prevented them fulfilling their devotional obligations. Those too weak to attend the chapel at St. Julian's were permitted to say their services where they were, and if too feeble even for that they were to "lie peacefully and say what they can". It was also accepted at both Sherburn and at Enköping that illness might prevent lepers attending services. Those, however, who without good reason neglected their devotions were punished. At St. Nicholas', Harbledown, public confession and castigation was arranged for defaulters and the omitted devotions were to be repeated in duplicate, as an errant schoolboy might have to write out in "lines" the work he has failed to learn.

The distinctive clothes mentioned in the general rules of conduct for lepers and described in detail in the regulations for several hospitals, have traditionally been seen as a warning of the danger of infection. The regulations of St. Julian's show them on the contrary to have been an outward sign of a religious and social outcast:

> "Since amongst all infirmities the disease of leprosy is held in contempt, those who are struck down with such a disease ought to show themselves only at special times and places, and in their manner and their dress more contemptible and humble than other men; as the Lord says in Leviticus, 'whosoever is disfigured with leprosy should wear his clothes open, his head bare, his mouth covered with a cloth, and call out that he is unclean and contaminated'." (7)

Unclean, contaminated, and contemptible—but no mention of infectious: for the individual, his dress marked him out as an outcast; to the institution, it was the uniform of membership which was different at each hospital. It is doubtful whether lepers isolated at home wore any distinctive dress.

The regulations of St. Julian's give a particularly clear description of its uniform: an ankle-length tunic of russet (a coarse reddish-brown cloth) with sleeves closed to the wrist "but not laced with threads in the secular fashion", a russet cowl and a cape of black cloth. Common dress changed little during the Middle Ages and lepers were no exception. A picture in a thirteenth-century French manuscript of a leper with clapper and begging bowl (Plate 16), and a marginal

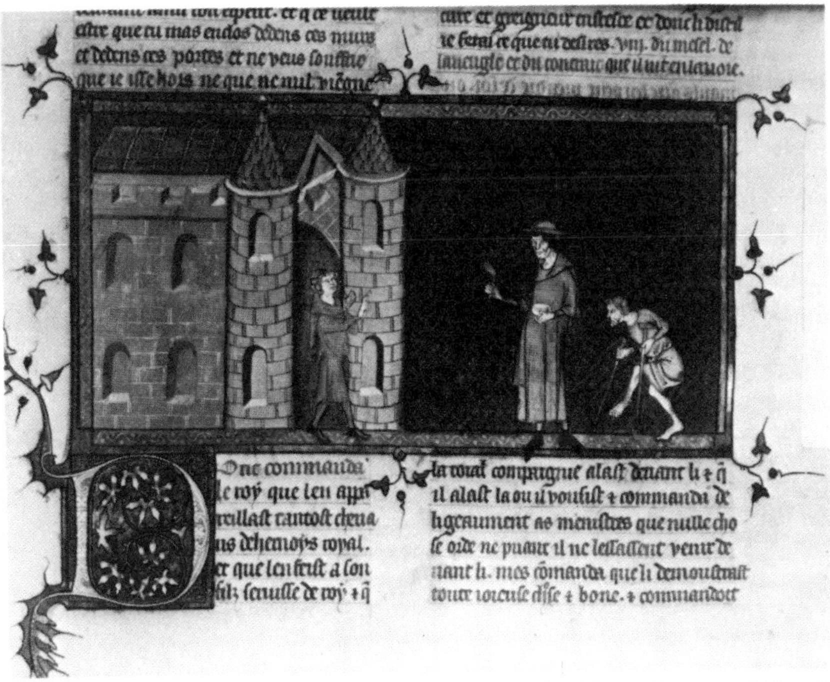

Plate 16. A leper with clapper and bowl: illustration in the thirteenth-century "Miroir Historial" of Vincent de Beauvais.

painting (Plate 15) of fourteenth- or fifteenth-century date in a manuscript of the Exeter Pontifical both show dress similar to the uniform of St. Julian's, apart from saucer-shaped hats which do not figure in any known regulations. The cloak of the English leper is russet and his hood black. It is worth noting, however, that although the French leper's outfit is longer than that of the man sending him away it is not otherwise very different from his.

Nor was there any great difference between the clothes of lepers and priests. The regulations of St. Julian's are just as detailed in respect to the habit of its priests as to the garments of its lepers. The priest's uniform was similar in character but different in colour: the tunic, cloak and hood were black, a style adopted also by priests at the sister house of St. Mary Prata near St. Albans. Their tunic must also reach the ankles and its sleeves extend to the back of the hand; their shoes, like those of the lepers, were described in detail and were deliberately unfashionable. Contrary to the popular tradition that there was one uniform to mark out all lepers as men apart, nothing suggests that deeper significance should be attached to the clothes of either lepers or priests at St. Julian's than to the uniform of any English school today. Regulation dress was not the prerogative of lepers: other types of hospital had their own uniform, such as the hospital of St. Cross at Winchester, which preserves its monkish habit to this day.

Two strange accidents of history confirm that lepers, priests, and people wore similar clothes. At about the same time that abbot Michael confirmed and revised the regulations of St. Julian's, a man was murdered in Halland on the south-west coast of Sweden by a heavy blow to the side of his head. His murderers, fearing that his spirit might torment them, buried him in a peat bog where the boundaries of four parishes met—a situation from which no spirit could escape. To make certainty doubly certain his murderers drove an oak stake through his heart and birch stakes through his back and side. He lay hidden there for nearly six hundred years until, in 1936, a farmer cutting peat at Bocksten found his body. The local policeman hastened to the spot, six centuries too late to solve the murder (8). The clothes of this fourteenth-century man (Plate 17) had been remarkably well preserved in the peat bog; apart from his trousers and fashionable "liripipe" extension to the hood of his cowl he might have been a leper dressed to the command of the abbot of St. Albans. Similar everyday clothes, with long tunic closed to the wrist and a cowl (Plate 18), were found in the frozen soil of the churchyard at Herjolfsnes in Greenland in 1921 (9). They enshrouded the remains of a man belonging to one of the last generations of the Norsemen on Greenland who, in the fifteenth century, disappeared without trace into the Arctic mists (10).

As time passed the old rules gradually assumed a new significance. The fourteenth-century regulations of Enköping leper hospital in Sweden insisted on strict isolation and warned of the danger that "the christian population is likely to become infected by *conversation and contact* with hospital patients". The Enköping regulations date from the period immediately after the Black Death, a cataclysm sufficient to stir the imagination to thoughts and fears of transmission of disease from one person to another. Nevertheless, awareness of the need to prevent the spread of leprosy antedated the Black Death. When the rules of St. Julian's hospital were revised shortly before the Black Death, they stipulated that the six leper-brothers should live apart from the healthy members of the institution "because of the risk of contagion". The gradual introduction of compulsory admission to a leper hospital, and changes in the punishment threatened to those who absconded, confirm a fundamental change in attitude towards leprosy during the Middle Ages.

Once admission to hospital had become compulsory, as for example at Enköping, expulsion ceased to be an appropriate punishment for misdemeanors. Minor offences continued to be punished by the customary loss of rations for a few days or weeks: at Exeter, for example, "if any brother or sister do in anger, malice or displeasure, strike or lay violent hands upon one the other, he shall be punished in the stocks, and have but bread and water for thirty days". Punishment by loss of rations long outlived the Middle Ages, and at Själö hospital in Finland in the seventeenth century anyone found guilty of "a fight resulting in breathlessness, hair-pulling, or getting blue and bloody" was to lose three months' rations. For persistent disobedience Enköping hospital threatened "an even worse punish-

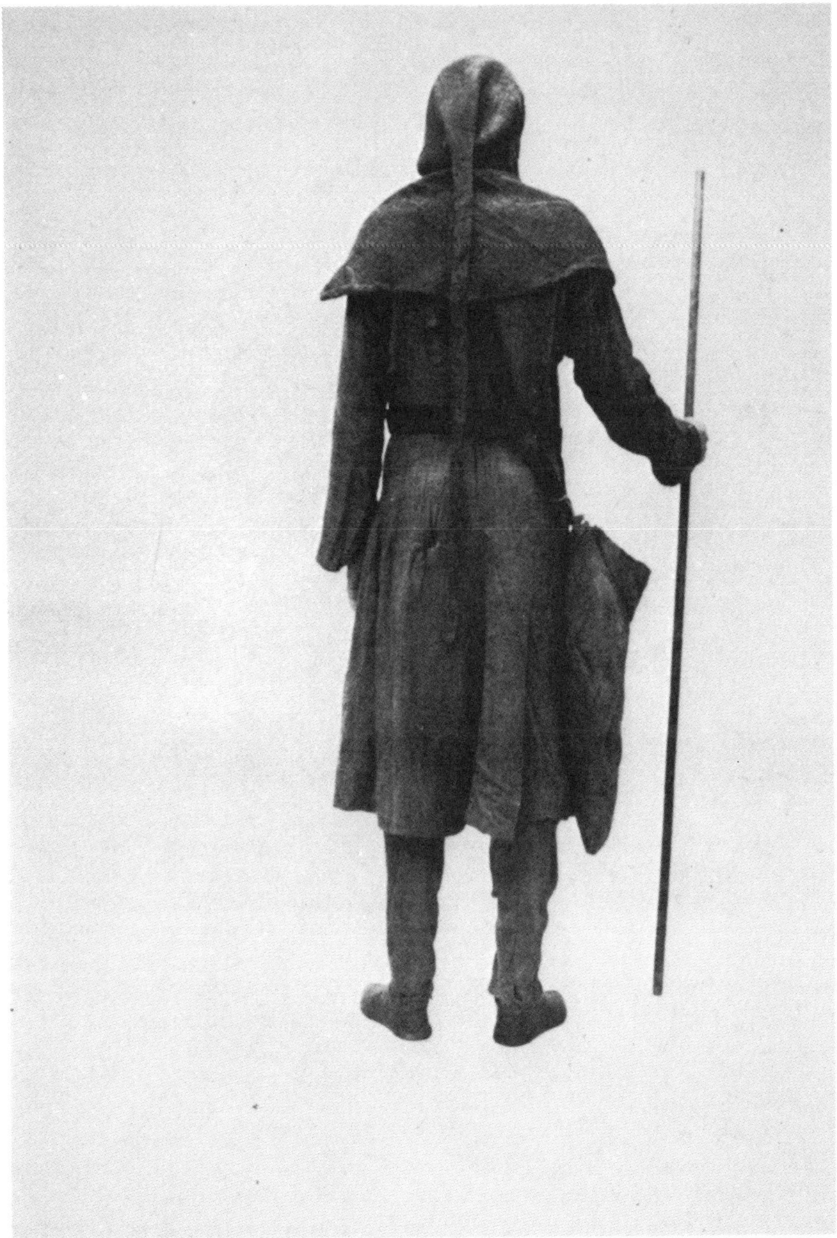

Plate 17. Clothing of the Bockstén man buried in a Swedish bog about 1360.

ment", but failed to define it. Perhaps it was the same as at Edinburgh in the late sixteenth century, where obedience was demanded "under the payne of hanging", no idle threat judged from the gallows set up beside the hospital—

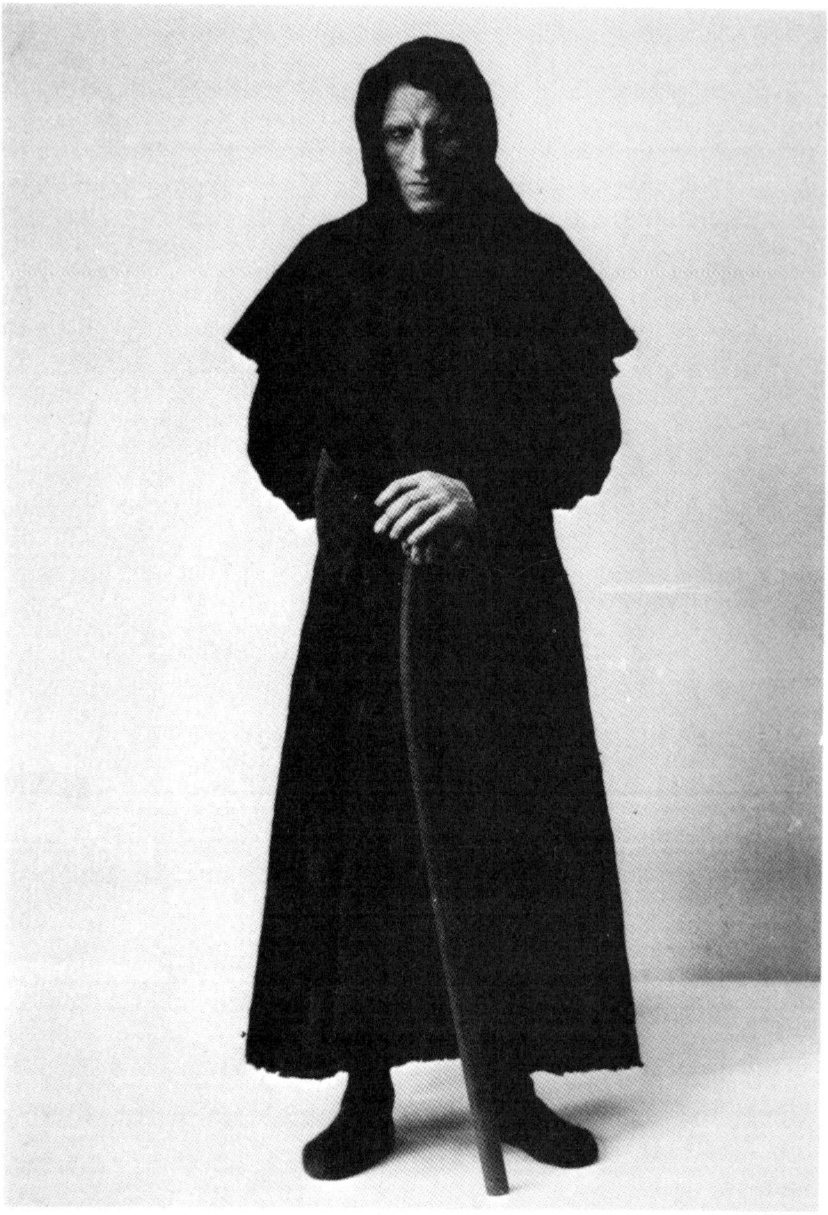

Plate 18. Clothing of a man buried in the frozen churchyard at Herjolfsnes, Greenland, about 1400.

"And thairfore, for the better obedience thairof, and for terrefying the said lepperis to transgress the samyn, the said commissioners has thocht meitt and expedient that there be ane gibbet sett up at the gavell of the said hospital." (11)

Yet, although the pulse of place and period can be taken, it is still not possible to weld fragmentary impressions into reliable generalisations. At almost the same time as Edinburgh erected its gallows the magistrates at Glasgow, no more than fifty miles away, stated that disobedience would be punished by "banishering" a leper from the hospital.

A gradual awareness that leprosy might be infectious also permeates the increasingly cautious regulations for visitors to hospitals. At Sherburn, permission was originally given for "their friends and well-wishers to visit and comfort them without hindrance and stay with them overnight, if they have come a long way and are rare visitors". Such licence would have struck terror into the suspicious heart of Abbot Michael of St. Albans, who (not for reasons of public health), strictly limited female visitors to "a mother or sister or honest matron", and then only at the "proper hour". Anyone whose female visitor overstayed was without further ado to be "punished as though guilty of unchastity", a vice of which the abbot clearly considered his disfigured flock capable because he deemed it necessary to prohibit "women of easy fame and low reputation" from entering the hospital. But as surely as infection was not seriously considered at St. Julian's and Sherburn at the time of their foundation in the twelfth century, the opposite was true of Enköping in the fourteenth century, where visitors were forbidden, as they were at Edinburgh two hundred years later. Practices varied, however, and at Exeter in the fifteenth century visitors were still allowed with the permission of the warden or his deputy.

However slowly the fear of infection became the most compelling reason for the isolation of lepers, it was probably dominant by the end of the fifteenth century. The chancery warrant concerning Joanna Nightingale refers to the "grievous injury and manifest perils . . . on account of the contagion of the aforesaid disease". In 1477, 1479, and again in 1481, "Andro Sauer" of Prestwick in Scotland was arraigned before the town's officials for visiting the nearby leper house at Kingcase. It was alleged that he was "abil to infect ye hale towne and weris ye seik folkis claithes and bonnettis". Again, however, a bewildering conflict of views is evident. One hundred years later, inmates of the Brigend hospital at Glasgow were allowed into the city provided they advertised their presence with their clappers and stood apart:

> "It is statut and ordanit that the Lipper of the hospital sall gang only on the calsie (street) syde near the gutter, and sall haif clapperis and ane claith upon their mouth and face, and sall stand afar of . . ." (12)

It is tempting to ascribe to the cloth over the mouth the function of a surgeon's mask, but it is much more likely only to represent fulfilment of the Levitical precept.

In contrast, a Danish law of 1522 insisted that the leper should stay outside the town:

> "So that common wayfaring men can recognise the leper he should have a wooden rattle and rattle with it. He should stand just outside the gate of the town. . . ." (13)

Prevention of infection was the explicit purpose of isolating lepers in seventeenth-century Finland. The royal patent of 1619 authorising the foundation of Själö hospital referred to the "infectious plague and disease of leprosy". And the meaning of the word infectious has not changed; one reason given for the increase in leprosy in Finland was that "those who are afflicted with it mix carelessly with those who are healthy and live among them". The logical decision was taken to build a hospital on a remote island "in order to separate these poor miserable people from the healthy". Even a person who had been in close contact with lepers was forbidden to "mix with other people *for at least one year*, so that it can be ascertained whether he is free of the disease or not", a precaution which reveals a remarkable awareness that the incubation period may be very long. Thirty-two years later, Per Brahe made it quite clear that the reason for founding a leper hospital on the Åland islands was to ensure that "this dangerous and infectious disease should not get completely out of hand". At the same time the twenty lepers in Gammelstad's hospital in Helsingfors were also referred to as having a "dangerous and infectious disease".

Fear of infection was not mere words. A 12-year-old boy, "Clement's son in Marby", was reported at Hammarland on Åland in 1648 to be "very careless and obeys no prohibition; he runs about amongst the children in the village to the sorrow and fear of the people". It was not only disobedient children who caused alarm and consternation: Muur made a note at Hammarland in January 1664 that "There are two lepers in Ekröö Torp who have been under observation for four years. ... The peasants maintain that the lepers are careless in mixing with the healthy, they take water from their wells, stride over stiles, live near the houses, walk boldly in and around the church amongst young people. Although they are forbidden such bold intercourse they take no notice. ..."

The purpose of isolation of the sick was to protect the healthy. Thus a leper who had retired to voluntary isolation sometimes pleaded successfully to be left alone because "there is no danger". For instance, it was reported at Lemland on February 23rd, 1640, that "Everyone thinks that the Finnish boy, Olle, is a leper; through a dispensation he was provided with shelter and food by the open water, and was given permission to walk to the gates of the farms during the day, provided he returned to his hovel in the evening." But solitary isolation of a sentenced leper was not common; to have a leper on the farm, even in a remote corner, was not good for business. Knut of Lemböte complained to the parish meeting at Lemland in 1642 that he could not hire labourers for his farm because they were frightened of his leprous brother who wandered around the fields. Not only were they afraid of being infected by meeting lepers, but even by touching objects they had handled. For this reason Erik of Norboda was in 1646 forbidden to make gloves for sale while he was under observation at home. Demand for his skill proved greater, however, than fear of his disease: he disobeyed the order and four years later the parish of Lemland had to declare once again that "From to day both men and women are forbidden to buy the gloves he used to sell, and nobody must let him make gloves from their hides."

Also in Finland, at Själö hospital nearly a century later, in 1725, a small gesture of personal sacrifice (of someone else) reveals that infection by leprosy was still feared. When the hospital had been rebuilt after the war between Sweden and Russia, and the church bells had been recovered from the chaplain who had deserted his post and fled to Sweden, the only place which could be found to hang the bells was a little belfry above the lepers' living-room. But who then was to run the leper gauntlet to ring the bell? Brita Rasmonsdotter, who had entered the hospital sixteen years previously with her leprous parents, was pressed into service. Her parents were now dead and she remained in the hospital not on account of leprosy but because "she was and still is of a weak brain". The authorities argued that because poor Brita was accustomed to live with lepers, she might as well continue to do so. She was forthwith "ordered to look after the sick people ... and cannot be allowed to be with the healthy. She, being the most healthy amongst the lepers, should in future see to the bell-ringing."

The most impressive evidence of the fear of infection was the burning of buildings which had housed lepers. When St. George's hospital in Åbo was closed in 1622 and the lepers were moved to Själö, the old hospital buildings were burnt "so that others shall not be infected with the same disease". An order was given at a meeting of the parish of Hammarland on the Åland islands in 1658 that "the lepers' houses in Posta and Bredhbolsta must be burned down".

Fear of infection was a relatively sophisticated concept, but plain, downright fear was another matter. A disfigured face or mutilated limb excites in most onlookers not only revulsion but also a primitive fear. Not necessarily fear of acquiring the same condition as in this case, but an instinctive fear of something horrible. Medieval physicians described the disfigurement of lepers as "frightful" and "satyr-like", and whatever the other reasons for removing a leper from the community it is very likely that dislike, horror, and fear underpinned them all.

This primitive fear was not particularly medieval, it was just human, and for that reason it lives on. Much is said in little in this regard by the dramatically simple yardstick of diagnosis recommended to the Åland parish of Lemland on March 9th, 1654: "Kirsten of Söderby was ordered to be inspected by the parish, and to be placed under observation *if they shudder at her.*" One hundred and sixty years later the reaction was just the same. Pastor Welhaven described how "a splendid fellow becomes as a leper insufferable in his peaceful neighbourhood ... both in church and in his house his company becomes repulsive ... if he even speaks to somebody in the street the other person turns away, for he finds his appearance offensive and repugnant". Even after fifteen years familiarity with the disease, Welhaven had to admit that "not without terror can it be met with in its severe forms".

A glance at some of Welhaven's parishioners and their successors (Plates 29–41) should convince the most hardened reader that at heart modern man is medieval and medieval modern; both are simply human.

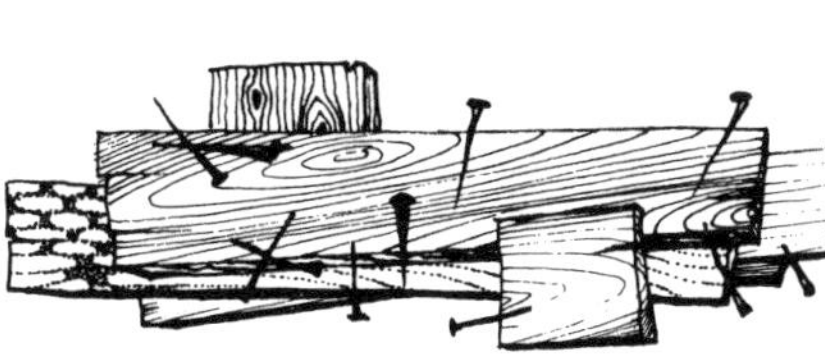

VII

Husbands and Wives

Few consequences of the disease were harder to bear, and none legally more tangled, than the long shadow it cast over the leper's marriage. What meaning had the vows of a person prevented by separation from fulfilling the obligations of marriage, one who no longer had the rights of other men under the law (1) and who, in the eyes of the Church, was dead to the world? Lawyers of both Church and State wrestled with the question throughout the Middle Ages and for long afterwards without finding a satisfactory answer.

A French law of 757 accepted leprosy as a cause for separation of husband and wife, if not divorce, and leprosy was included in Welsh laws of the tenth to twelfth centuries, along with "foul breath" and failure to have sexual relations, as a legitimate cause for a wife to leave her husband and reclaim her dowry. An eleventh-century Norwegian law declared that a promise of marriage was not binding if one of the partners was found to be a leper, a view shared by the Roman Church. In 1186 Pope Urban III decreed that

> "Betrothal cannot compel people to get married if leprosy occurs between the time of betrothal and the proposed marriage" (2)

—a theme continued in Denmark as recently as 1922, when leprosy concealed before marriage was held to be valid grounds for divorce. In the view of the medieval Church expressed by Pope Alexander III, leprosy did not debar a person from marriage provided a willing partner could be found—

> "... if lepers do not wish to remain continent, and they find someone willing to marry them, they are allowed to enter matrimony" (2)

Those unfortunate enough to find themselves married to someone who subsequently developed leprosy were exhorted to long-suffering. In a letter to the Archbishop of Canterbury in 1180, Pope Alexander III stated that leprosy was not valid grounds for divorce:

> "We command that you should not delay in strongly persuading wives to follow husbands and husbands to follow wives who have contracted leprosy and to care for them with conjugal love. But if they cannot be persuaded to do this you should strictly order them to observe continence whilst either of them is alive. And if they refuse to accept your order, you should excommunicate them." (2)

But admission to hospital changed everything between husband and wife. For a start, the monastic rules of medieval leper hospitals insisted upon chastity. Secondly, as at St. Julian's for example, a married man was admitted only if his wife also took religious vows or if she "was of such an age that she can remain in the world without suspicion of incontinence, and both she and her husband have made a vow of perpetual chastity before the archdeacon". In practice it was not quite so easy; for instance, an assize roll of 1254 records that Amicia, a woman of Kent, attempted to marry again but was forced to confess that her former husband, a leper in Romney hospital, was still alive. The reasoning behind this regulation was simple and widely accepted: the partners must agree because "man and wife are made one flesh in married union, and it is not possible for one part to turn to the Lord and the other to remain in the world". The impossibility was part philosophical and part physical, particularly the latter because, as the St. Julian's regulations explained, "if the sick spouse demands payment from his or her body then, according to the general teaching of the Apostle, what is due must be paid".

Some leper foundations were restricted to men and a few to women, but many admitted both. It was thus possible for husband and wife to seek admission to the same hospital, if they were both lepers, as a couple did at St. Margaret's hospital at Huntingdon in 1327. The St. Julian's regulations made it clear, however, that they would not be able to live as husband and wife in the hospital and at Sherburn too the "brothers" and "sisters" lived apart, although they attended church services together. The women were supervised by their own prioress. Although they lived apart, the "brothers" and "sisters" were expected to work together—at least in Sweden and Finland: at Enköping in Sweden they were expected to join in the hay-making and harvesting together, and three centuries later Själö hospital in Finland required any "who have the strength and ability" to "help with the hay and harvest as well as to row off to milk, and help with all the tasks of use to the hospital; in the winter they must not refuse to make fishing nets". Later in the Middle Ages, in Denmark in particular, healthy individuals including close relatives were admitted to leper hospitals to help with the day-to-day work, as has been discussed, but they almost certainly lived apart.

For the wife of a leper her husband's admission to hospital relieved her of the burden of looking after him at the expense not only of self-imposed chastity, but also of the loss of part or, in some places, of all her inheritance from him. Conversely, where the wife was the leper, her admission to hospital deprived her husband of her dowry. If a leper lived outside hospital and received no support from it he could dispose of his property as he pleased. Once admitted to hospital, and regardless of whether or not he made a payment on admission, he was obliged to bequeath part or all of his possessions to the hospital. One of the first things a leper was expected to do on admission to St. Julian's was to make an inventory of his possessions and to make a will. Up to one third of the possessions brought with him into hospital might be left to whom he chose, but the residue was to be used for the benefit of the hospital and its inmates. This enforced bequest to the hospital was not peculiar to lepers; the clerics belonging to the hospital were required to "follow the same rule and method" in making their own wills. In practice, the only difference was that the clerics were not obliged to remain in the hospital for the rest of their days. In England, the rule that a leper must bequeath part of his property to the institution which sheltered him continued into the fifteenth century at least. A parchment roll of 1449–50 at Totnes in Devon records that "every brother or sister, a leper, entering the house of St. Mary Magdalene shall at the end of his or her life leave there in the custody of the wardens one bed, one platter, one pot towards the support of the house and its chaplain, unless so poor as not to be possessed of such goods".

Further north, as the regulations of Enköping hospital show, greater demands were made upon the lepers' possessions. Not only were they required, and if necessary compelled ("both they or their heirs") to bring all their moveable possessions to the hospital "to be used for the common good", but their other assets were categorised as "goods given or bequeathed to churches and other holy places"; in short all that they possessed now belonged to the hospital, and the widow could expect nothing. There was no need even to wait for a will to be proved; this bequest needed no will. All the possessions a leper took with him into Svendborg hospital in Denmark also passed to the hospital for general use on his death, but no mention was made of his other property.

Once again, it is the survival of the same practice on Åland which makes these medieval regulations credible. Three hundred years after the Enköping regulations were written, Anna of Månstekta died at home after several years under observation for suspected leprosy. She was never admitted to hospital, but after her death the parish meeting at Sund on January 27th, 1656, ordered an enquiry into her estate: "all the articles must be valued and they belong to the hospital". At another meeting a few days later it was resolved that "The situation should be clarified concerning the outstanding estate of the leper Anna which was to be demanded from her brother's sister, also the remaining 14 daler which Per Sefferson sent to the late sheriff." Anna's obligation to the hospital, and it is likely that the same was true of Erik of Norboda in a similar case, probably arose from the acceptance of alms or "Christmas fare" during her isolation at home which would otherwise have gone to the hospital; whatever the reason, it is clear that the property of both of them was considered to belong to the hospital, and that pressure was exerted on the next of kin to recover it. Erik's diagnosis was confirmed by the parish in 1652 after several years of home isolation; he was sentenced to be taken away to hospital, but seems to have died before he was moved. The parish meeting at Lumparland on August 19th, 1654 was told that "the widow of the late Erik has carried her late husband's clothes down to the lake. As she was not present instructions were given about his clothes and his house." Perhaps by putting his clothes out for collection she had optimistically hoped they would not press their claim to possession of her home.

After the Reformation, monasticism no longer simplified the relationship between husband and wife. The legal situation was particularly complicated when they mutually agreed on a permanent separation. In 1658, the cathedral chapter of Åbo refused a divorce to a man in Kuhmo who had entered into an adulterous relationship during the seven years his wife had been in a leper hospital; possibly he argued that even if leprosy was no pretext for divorce, adultery was. Instead of a divorce he was exhorted to bear his "cross with patience and pray God to enable him to do so with a good spirit until God calls her ... and who knows, God can call her soon enough". The following year, Matts Simonson of Harjavalta, whose wife was a leper in Själö hospital, was more successful with his petition. He had already "besieged" a certain woman for the second time and wished to marry her. The chapter asked him first to visit the hospital to discover whether or not his wife was still alive and, if so, to seek her permission to marry again. This Matts firmly refused to do. Eventually the chapter pragmatically resolved that it "was better to admit him to marriage", but insisted that the couple must not be married in their own community, and that they must undertake to move away to a place where neither of them was known. He may have relented and visited his leprous wife after all, because the following year a woman patient at Själö gave her husband permission to re-marry. The cathedral chapter clearly accepted the realities of the situation, but at the same time wanted no publicity for their controversial decision. They were not alone in their realistic approach, for at Helsingfors in 1661 a man called Eric Göransson, whose wife had been in hospital with leprosy for nine years, was allowed to marry again.

The most fascinating episode of the marriage saga took place at Åbo on December 15th, 1673, when the chapter met to consider a request by the wife of a leper in Själö hospital to take another husband. It proved to be one thing for the husband of a leper to re-marry, but quite another for the wife of a leper to take the same step. Her legal husband, Hans Mattson, a farmer, had been in the leper hospital since New Year's day, 1669, and his wife knowing full well that he would never come home again had asked her pastor at Björneborg whether, with her husband's full consent, she could now marry a boatman who had proposed to her. The pastor referred the thorny question to the cathedral chapter at Åbo and an eyewitness's account of their deliberations has survived (3).

First, Tammelinus, headmaster of the cathedral school arose to speak. With caution appropriate for one who was not only out of his depth but in the presence of his employers, he hedged; he said that he would prefer to refer the matter for the consideration of others, although personally he was not opposed to the marriage if the highest ecclesiastical court in the country was prepared to grant a dispensation. Tunander, a professor of theology, now made the following observations: first, her husband had no hope of recovery from leprosy; second, God had himself separated them and the man was now dead to the world; third, leprosy is a unique disease and lepers must according to the old testament be segregated; fourth, she had already waited a long time; fifth, her husband had given his permission for her to marry again. Clearly he supported the petition, but he did not actually nail his colours to the mast. Bång, another professor of theology now struggled to his feet and, as a rival professor in a small university often will, adopted a contrary opinion. In his view, marriage was a mysterious relationship both morally and physically, and this fact was in no way altered by leprosy. He argued that the old testament expressed a contrary view to that of his colleague, and he noted that Christ compared his own relationship with the church to matrimony and did not lightly consent to divorce. Finally, he made the outrageous remark that the woman did not suffer great hardship because, after all, she only wished to marry a boatman. He considered that she should not marry another as long as her husband lived. Enewaldus, dean of the cathedral and a Swede by birth, was then called upon for his opinion. He said that because marriage was a religious mystery it was not wholly according to his conscience to separate them; in his opinion the matter should be deferred until parliament reassembled—not an entirely logical conclusion one feels, but diplomatic because his chief, the bishop, had yet to speak. Bishop John Gezelius the elder (Plate 19) finally spoke. Such a marriage was not "nowadays" permitted, he said, nevertheless he had heard of two similar cases in the country of Nyland recently, and he undertook to examine the circumstances and precedents of those cases when he next made an inspection visit there. The chapter resolved that a letter should be sent to the pastor of Björneborg instructing him to persuade the woman not to marry another man, but to

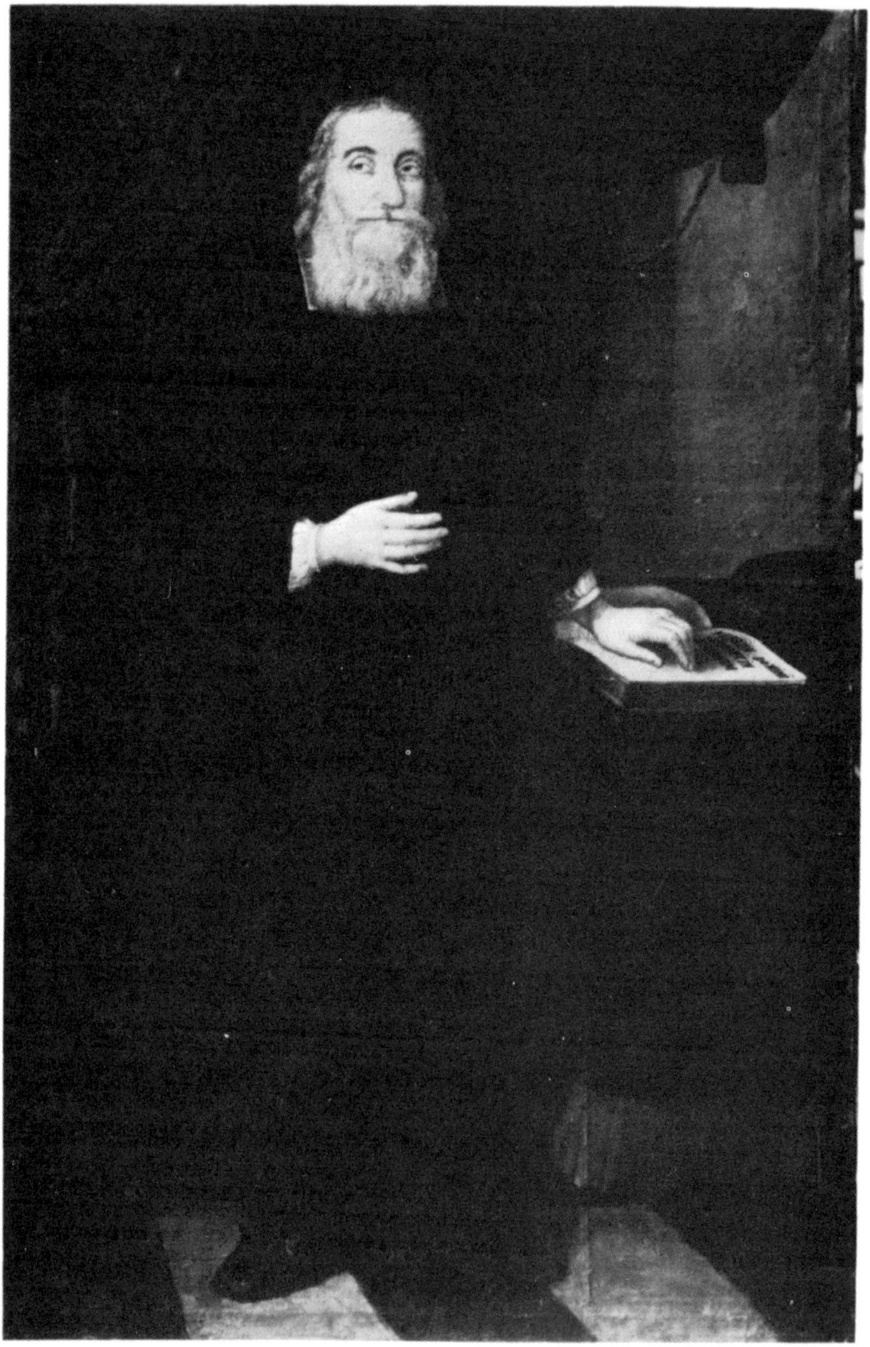

Plate 19. Bishop Gezelius the elder, who in 1673 presided over the cathedral chapter of Åbo when they considered whether the wife of a leper in hospital might marry again, with her husband's permission, while he still lived.

remain chaste. The voting for this motion is not recorded; at a guess, the bishop, respectful dean, and Bång were for it, Tunander against, and Tammelinus a cautious abstention. Not for six long years did Hans Mattson die. Whether the boatman still waited patiently for his wife will never be known.

Bishop Gezelius was succeeded on his death in 1690 by his son. His father's verdict in the case of Hans Mattson's wife had clearly disturbed him, for in 1693 he sent a memorandum to the cathedral chapter on the annulment of a leper's marriage. In his opinion, the healthy partner "had on his side all that God's word had to say about the use and purpose of marriage": their physical separation was so complete that, as far as the healthy spouse and her children were concerned, the leprous partner might as well be dead. He also thought it possible to interpret "the law" to say that no one could be bound to support in marriage an infirm or "for the purposes of marriage, utterly useless partner". He further maintained that the shattered marriage not only caused domestic hardship and neglect of the children's upbringing, but the deterioration of the family's business affairs. Finally, he decided that those theologians who refused the request for re-marriage were under the misapprehension that the healthy spouse continued to live together with the leprous partner. After long and careful consideration his compassionate conclusion was that "it seemed hard to deny a divorce to the healthy partner of the marriage". In spite of the new bishop's attitude a divorce remained difficult to obtain: in 1705, a farmer, Carl Hindriksson, found it necessary to petition the king for a divorce from his wife Maria who had been admitted to Kronoby hospital with leprosy.

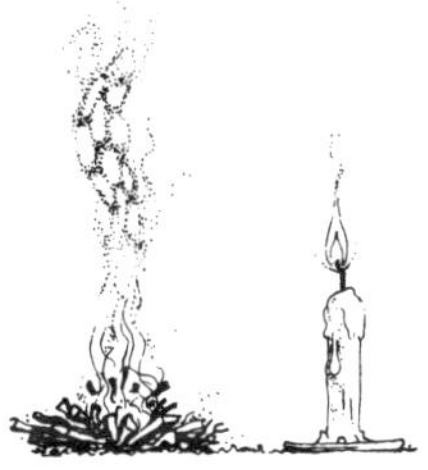

VIII

Despair and Hope

Hunger, cold, and the loss of family, friends, and home were only one aspect of a leper's suffering. Heaviest of all his burdens was omnipresent death, a fate not hidden from him, a companionship sometimes both long and painfully drawn out. Death was the central theme of the church service which formally removed him from the medieval world. His life henceforth was indeed "a living death", as Welhaven described it in Bergen in the nineteenth century, until time sooner or later conferred finality upon it.

The form of the service is precisely recorded (1) and with a minimum of licence the scene can be recreated. The place could as well be Salisbury in England, Bergen in Norway, Åbo in Finland or, indeed, any other European city, for the Church imposed a uniformity of practice careless of national frontiers. The date could be any time between 1200 and 1400; time moved very slowly. Even as we watch, the bustle in the busy street stops, its clatter and chatter fades away. The glint of sunlight on a silver cross catches our attention as a silent little procession comes slowly into sight: a bearer holding high a cross, a robed priest and, last of all, a curiously and horribly disfigured man, limping a little, his head bowed, and his eyes cast down. The bystanders know him well as one of themselves, but for many months past they have seen little of him. Last year people were whispering about him: they said his face was becoming dusky red and lumpy; his voice was becoming hoarse and harsh. In church nobody would stand close to him, and fewer and fewer people bought the gloves he made. Gradually, sensing their accusing glances and whispers, he had withdrawn from their company. Now they know that their suspicions were well-founded, for only one disease slowly devours and disfigures a man like this: he is a leper. For a moment the townsfolk pause, with as much or as little respect as a passing funeral commands — a shrug of the shoulders, a brief second's thought — then the world revolves again, and the day's work continues.

The world revolved again, but their world is his no longer. In the church a black cloth is draped over two trestles before the altar; under this pall the leper kneels, hears mass, and makes his last confession. The service said, the priest casts a sprinkling of earth over his feet, as if into the open grave, and solemnly commands him to be dead to the world but alive again to God.

Draped with that same black cloth, his living shroud, the leper moves to the door of the church where he pauses for a moment while the priest sprinkles him with holy water, and commends him to the none-too-loving care of the people. Cross, priest and leper progress once more. Soon we lose sight of them and turn back towards the clatter of carts, hubbub of voices and all the hustle and bustle of the town. Behind us a faint chant is carried clearly on the wind "*Libera me Domine*", fainter and fainter still, "*Libera me* ..." as the priest precedes the leper to his place of isolation as if he were a funeral bier. In the hospital his last frail strands of hope part when confronted with the rule that he must quickly make his last will and testament. The small codicil that the document was to be returned to him "if he should recover" must have seemed a prospect too forlorn to cherish. "Remember thine end and thou shalt never do amiss" the priest had said in the service of seclusion—how could the poor leper forget it?

The special service for lepers died as the Reformation was born, but the message of its pall and scattered earth was not extinguished. Inevitable and imminent death stared the lepers of seventeenth-century Åland in the face with a force and candour unequalled even in the Middle Ages. One new requirement was added to the every-day goods and chattels lepers had for centuries brought with them into hospital—wood and nails for their own coffins. This item appears for the first time in a resolution of Muur's own parish of Saltvik on March 10th, 1658, in these words:

> "Maths Bengtson of Fremanby and Erich Hanson of Ökarby are instructed to make ready clothes of all sorts for several years use. Also bedclothes, wood and nails for coffins, axe, cooking pots, drinking and eating utensils ... so that these sick people can be taken away in the Spring as soon as the crops have been sown." (2)

Maths Bengtson never reached the hospital; Erich Hanson was admitted on September 7th and died sometime between 1661 and 1664. Even two small leper children reported to a meeting of the parish of Hammarland in 1658 were provided with wood and nails for their own coffins. In this requirement, as in many others, the parishes often fell short, so much so that in 1664 they were threatened with fines if again "contrary to the dean's instructions the lepers have not brought with them beer barrels, drinking vessels and coffins. ..."

The leper could no more forget his fate than he could escape it. Many and various penalties were devised in the Middle Ages to persuade lepers to obey writs for their exclusion. London threatened a baker, John Mayne, with the pillory in 1372 if he returned to the city. Bristol punished lepers who would not leave the city by imprisonment. Berwick-on-Tweed threatened worse penalties: the statutes of the Society of Merchants of Berwick, drawn up by the mayor in 1283–84, stated that "If one wilfully forces his way in, his clothes shall be taken off him and burnt, and he shall be turned out naked." In mitigation of this harsh measure the statutes continued "for we have already taken care that a proper place for lepers shall be kept up outside the town and that alms shall there be given to them". Regulations gradually became stricter everywhere. In Copenhagen, a stutute of 1443 (subsequently applied to the whole of Denmark by King Hans) stated that "Whosoever in the town catches leprosy must go to St. George's hospital within the period that the sheriff and mayor allow him. If he does not do so, they must take him and his possessions."

The Middle Ages passed, but much that was medieval remained. At Edinburgh in 1530, *De leproso amovendo* reappeared in its Scottish version *Anent Lipper Folke*, with a more than medieval ferocity. The law declared that "no manner of Lipper persone, man nor woman, fra this tyme forth, cum amangis uther cleine personis, nor be nocht fund in the kirk, fishe merket, nor fleshe merket, nor no other merket within this burghe, under the payne of burnyng of their cheik and bannasing off the toune" (3). Nearly one hundred and fifty years later in Finland, the principle was the same, but the practice less cruel. The Governor of Åbo, Harold Oxe, wrote to the warden of Själö leper hospital on November 10th, 1670, concerning a leper who had persistently evaded an order to go to the hospital, saying

> "Although, Oluf Hendhersson, I have repeatedly advised you that Nills Rosenkrantz of Hallkilais in Pemar parish should present himself for admission to hospital he had done no such thing and can easily infect his brothers and sisters with whom he daily lives. In order to force him to comply with the order made against him the alderman and six of the strongest men who are themselves lepers should be sent there by boat to take him from his farm by force. If anyone tries to prevent them they are to take no notice, but carry out their task, and in due course report those who tried to hinder them and they will be punished later." (4)

He was admitted to Själö hospital on December 1st, 1670, and died there four months later to the day.

Rosenkrantz was not the only one forced to enter hospital. Ten years previously the Governor of Åbo had ordered that a woman in Kimito should be taken by force to Själö hospital. She had been confirmed to be "leprous and infectious" but absolutely refused to leave her home and family. On another occasion firm pressure was exerted on a leper's relatives to make sure that he went to hospital. In 1654 the district court of Lappua had decided that if a farmer whose wife had leprosy continued in his refusal to send her to hospital, his house should be pulled down without further argument; any parishioners who helped or harboured lepers were liable to be fined.

Besides living with death a leper laboured under an undeserved imputation of guilt. A complex, ancient and widespread tradition equated leprosy with divine punishment of moral depravity (5). In Finland in 1440, "leprosy money" was paid to those "whom God pleases to *punish* with the disease of leprosy", and the royal foundation charter for Själö hospital in 1619 refers to "leprosy, which is a divine punishment *for sin*". Peder Olsen Feidie, who was himself admitted to St. George's leper hospital in Bergen in 1832, reveals in a unique, if rustic, poem (6) that this slur of divine punishment for sin—committed or uncommited—was still felt at the dawn of scientific medicine.

"Now after Jesus we must call—
O Lord have mercy on us all—
As the woman once cried.
This is our *punishment for sin*
therefore we cannot hope to win
More than a few small crumbs
Of mercy from thy grace."

A leper must also have been keenly aware that he was looked upon more with contempt than with compassion. He was estranged from God and cut off from his fellow men. The regulations of St. Julian's put his position in a nutshell:

> "Since amongst all infirmities the disease of leprosy is held in contempt, those who are struck down with such a disease ought to show themselves only at special times and places, and in their manner and dress more contemptible than other men". (7)

The accusation that Nicholas Harris, footpostman of Totnes, was "an uncleane manne and a Leaper, not fitte to come or be admitted into the company of cleane persons" bears witness five centuries later to the enduring stigma associated with leprosy; men's minds had failed to evolve with their surroundings.

More than this, his disfigurement made a leper doubly unacceptable and more profoundly isolated than separation alone could ever achieve. Welhaven poignantly expressed from his own experience the depth of a leper's isolation:

> "Separated from his former friends and acquaintances, plucked from the family circle and his rural occupations he is conveyed with his 'sick pass' to the town, to see himself in a terrifying mirror, to enter the company of other sufferers and to battle with want, suffering and depression. His longing naturally matches his suffering and becomes very deep as his disease makes him feel ever more isolated. He cannot look forward to many visits and even if he speaks to someone on the street the other person gives way, finding his appearance offensive and repugnant. Because of this he loses hope and so his misfortune is complete. ... The wretched leper ... must renounce the best of an individual's freedom and rights. Happiness flees him as well as life itself, and only death's certain call can comfort and satisfy him." (8)

Thus guilt and rejection ended in despair, despair compounded by the long drawn out clarion of "death's certain call".

Everyone, the leper most of all, knew that leprosy was incurable; to deny the fact was tantamount to witchcraft. At the trial of Christian Livingston as a witch in Edinburgh in 1597 it was alleged that she "afirmit that she culd hail (cure) leprosie, quhilk the maist expert men in medicine are not able to do". For treatment she had taken "a reid cock, slew it, baked a bannock with the blude of it, and gif the samyn to the Leper to eat", a no more unreasonable and heretical recipe than a traditional Scottish remedy of the time, which claimed that "the blood of dogs and of infants two years old and under, when diffused through a bath of heated water dispels the Leprosy without a doubt".

No attempted treatment had a more dramatic and tragic outcome than at Elgin in Scotland at about this time. An eyewitness account has survived in the city archives but the date is not recorded. The townsfolk had decided that a certain Marjory Bysseth was a witch, and her final undoing was the result of testimony from a supposed leper whom she had kindly and freely tried to heal. The story cannot be better told than by the man who saw with his own eyes her trial, first by the mob and then in the waters of the ordeal pool.

> "... ane grete multitude rushinge through the Pannis port (Elgin) surroundit ye order (ordeal) pool and hither was draggit Marjory Bysseth, in sore plight, with her grey haires hanging loose, and crying 'Pitie! Pitie!' Now Maister Wiseman, the samin clerk, who had stode up at her tryal, stepped forward and saide 'I kno this womyan to have been ane peacable and unoffendyge ane, living in ye privacy of her widowhoode, and skaithing or gainsaying no one. Quhat have ye furthir to say again her?'
>
> Then did ye Friaries (friars) agen repeate how that she had muttered her Aves backward, and othirs that ye maukin (hare) started at Bareflet had been traced to her dwellinge, and how that the aforesaid cattal had died by her

connivance. Bot she hearing this cried the more 'Pitie! Pitie! I am guiltless of ye fausse crymes, never sae much as though of be mie.'

Then suddenly there was ane motion in ye crowd, and ye peopel parting on ilk syde, ane Leper came down frae ye Hous (the leper house) and in ye face of ye peopel bared his hand and his haill arm, ye which was wythered and covered over with scurfs, most piteous to behold, and he said 'At ye day of Pentecost last past, thys womyan did give unto me ane shell of oyntment, with ye which I annoynted my hand to cure ane imposthume which had cum over it, and behold from that day furthe untyll thys, it hath shrunk and wythered as you see it now.'"

The nature of his disease is obscure and unlikely to have been leprosy, but the medical uncertainty in no way detracts from the insight into the psychology of the times. Events now moved fast, and no protestations from honest clerk Wiseman could restrain the roused mob from demanding a trial by ordeal.

"Whereupon ye crowde closed rounde and becam clamorous: but ye said Marjory Bysseth cried piteously that God had forsaken her—that she had meanyed gude and not evil — that the oyntment was ane gift of her husband, who had been beyond the seas and that it was ane gift to him from ane holy man and true, and that she had given it free of reward or hyre, wishing only that it mote be of gude. ...

Whereupon the peopel did presse roun and becam clamorous and they tak ye womyan and drag her, amid mony tears and cryes to ye pool and crie 'To trial! To trial!' and soe they plonge her in ye water. And quhen she went down in ye water there was ane gret shoute; bot as she rose agayne and raised up her arms, as gif she wod have com up, there was a silence for ane space, when agane she gaed downe with ane bubblinge noise, and they shouted finallie—'to Sathan's Kingdom she hath gane' and forthwith went their wayes." (9)

Poor, innocent Marjory!

For centuries the disease continued to be incurable. On the Shetland Isles in 1735 the Rev. Andrew Fisken wrote that "none ever recovered", indeed the disease progressed inexorably until the face of the unhappy person resembled "a lump of rotten cork", an image which was also used by one of the Icelandic names of the disease—*likprar*, which Petersen in 1769 translated into Danish as "rotten corpse". Welhaven, early in the next century, had no illusions about the hopelessness of the disease, saying "I know for certain that all attempts to check and to eradicate this disease hitherto have been completely fruitless, even sometimes harmful to the patient." At about the same time a British doctor, Dr. Holland, touring Iceland referred to the three hospitals in which "a few incurable lepers receive gratuitous support" and commented that "when it is considered how frequently unsuccessful the treatment of this disease is in more auspicious regions it will not excite surprise that in Iceland the attempt at cure should generally be unavailing".

There was no cure—but it was only human to hope. By the nineteenth century witches had metamorphosed into "wise-women", like Lucia Pytter of Sandviken, who dignified herself with the title of "Madame" and advertised publicly in Bergen in 1804 that she was able to cure leprosy. Two leper girls were "loaned" to her from St. George's hospital so that she with "all possible diligence, good charge and care" might substantiate her claim. Welhaven recorded that "what Madame Pytter used for these sick girls is unknown to me, but after some weeks they both returned as wretched as before and died the same year with many afflictions and lesions". Two other lepers from Bergen were later sent to "Mother" Seather in Christiana (Oslo) for treatment, with an equally unimpressive result.

However ineffective the treatment given by these old women, their treatment was no less effective, and possibly less harmful, than contemporary medical treatment. A truly heroic trial by therapeutic ordeal began in Jarnuary 1774 at the Royal Seraphimer Hospital in Stockholm under the supervision of J. L. Odhelius, who had been physician at the hospital for twelve years. He had previously attempted treatment with many concoctions of herbs, shrubs, and trees used in different parts of Sweden without success. Then a Dr. Lyman of Torneå in the north of Sweden recommended an infusion of a strong concoction of juniper wood; when Odhelius found it to be useless, Lyman recalled that several other plants had been included in his mixture, one of which was *Ledum palustre*, bog myrtle. With a crusading spirit familiar to all doctors with the latest remedy in their hands, Odhelius writes that "I had just then a new patient with leprosy, and decided at once to make an experiment upon her." (10)

Thus on January 9th, Brita Söderberg, a 30-year-old woman, started to imbibe "as much as she was able to endure" of the "beautiful reddish-orange" liquid with "a slightly unpleasant taste" (more unpleasant no doubt in the opinion of the patient who had to take it than in the opinion of the doctor who dispensed it). "The first effect was headache, with giddiness and heat over the whole body, and when she drank too much or too fast, she vomited, but otherwise this fever was always followed by sweating." Within the dramatically short space of three days her leprous nodules appeared to soften and diminish, so much so that on January 14th, buoyed up with "joy over hope of improvement", she drank sufficient of her medicine "to heat her blood to the height that a blood-letting was necessary. She was warned to drink less and to await her improvement with patience." Odhelius must have felt that fame was just around the corner.

During the first month of treatment her leprous nodules continued to subside, and her ulcers started to heal, but, on February 26th, treatment had to be interrupted because she was "seized with violent vomiting, much enervation and giddiness". Instead, she began to wash herself all over with the medicine, but her strength was waning and "restorative measures" including creamy milk were introduced. By March 12th she had recovered sufficiently to start drinking the medicine again. Gradually she improved until, on May 29th, her legs began to swell and were treated, inappropriately one fears, with *mixtura salina riverii*. June 7th was punctuated by severe bloody diarrhoea culminating in the expulsion of a worm fully one foot long.

Fever, prostration, thirst, and dryness in the throat now returned and were treated with rhubarb, *spiritus vitrioli*, and a stomach plaster, with the later addition of *nux vomica*. By early July she had improved but still "her strength would not return". Odhelius relates proudly that "leprosy seemed much lessened", but adds regretfully that "no matter what means were used there appeared little hope of recovery of her health, and she died peacefully on July 31st". As has happened before and since, the doctor was convinced his treatment was a success only the patient died. His conviction was strengthened by the confession of her nurse that his patient had "secretly exchanged her milk and meat soup for herring and salt fish, and she drank cold water excessively. He presented the case before the Royal Swedish Academy of Science in the hope that others would test this treatment on less advanced cases.

Odhelius mentioned that he had previously tried treatment with mercury without success. The fact that mercury, in the form of quicksilver, was also used to treat syphilis is not evidence of confusion between the two diseases. Penicillin was also used indiscriminately when first introduced, but doctors were well able to distinguish between the many infectious diseases for which it was tried. Both Odhelius and Uddman in Sweden, and Petersen in Iceland, agreed that mercury was useless for leprosy, but all other treatments were equally ineffective. Should the doctor do nothing and admit his therapeutic impotence?

Several priests gave mercurial medicines to their leprous parishioners. Strøm pastor of the country parish of Bolden in west Norway in the seventeen sixties and seventies, dispensed mercurial brandy "with good effect", an effect doubtless no more profound than that of brandy itself upon morale! Treatment with mercury had been less than satisfactory on the Shetland Isles according to the Rev. Andrew Fisken who wrote in 1736 that "There has never been any cure of this disease attempted here, save that a few years ago a young woman in a neighbouring parish had some bolusses of mercury ... but some dangerous symptoms appearing, the administrator thought fit to proceed no further." (11)

Strøm also gave concoctions of antimony and juniper, the latter being a standard treatment both in Norway and in Iceland, where it was mentioned by Petersen in his monograph of 1769. The leprous priest who wrote to Petersen describing his symptoms had already been treated with juniper baths amongst other remedies, including leeches. Little had the lepers of Gloskär realised when they stripped the juniper bushes from outlying islands in their search for firewood that they were destroying a popular remedy for their disease. However, even if they had known, they would have been wiser to take the immediate comfort of its conflagration than to speculate upon its dubious medicinal properties. Besides juniper concoctions and baths, the Icelanders also used volcanic mudbaths and warm mineral water baths as treatment for leprosy and various skin diseases. Viper potions, a remedy for leprosy dating back to classical antiquity, were still known in eighteenth-century Sweden. Uddman mentioned them only to warn his readers that they were ineffective, not least, he suggested, because the common Swedish viper was a different species to the viper of classical antiquity. Nevertheless he did not entirely dismiss such remedies; on the contrary, he reproduced the formula of the latest viper and mercury potion from Edinburgh.

Of all medicinal treatments, well-water was probably the safest. Traditions of healing springs are as old as civilisation itself, and leprosy became caught up in these legends. Harbledown leper hospital near Canterbury was situated close to a spring long considered to have healing properties. So famous was the healing potency of this spring that the Black Prince sent for its waters in his last illness in 1376. Pastor Strøm in west Norway included well-water amongst the many remedies he energetically dispensed to the few lepers in his parish. He extolled its virtues in the treatment of a 30-year-old leper called T. Brune who, in 1773, developed additional symptoms of "depression, fantasies, and insomnia". In response to "two pots or more of vicarage well-water daily for eighteen days and a powder each evening, he lost his fantasies and his sleep improved". Alas, his signs of leprosy relentlessly progressed.

It was in Finland that treatment of leprosy with well-water achieved its greatest fame. In 1688, Elias Tillandz, professor of medicine at Åbo, investigated the healing properties of water from the nearby St. Henry's well at Kuppis. St. Henry was Bishop Henry the Englishman, who as Bishop of Uppsala, christianised Finland with bible and sword in 1155. A diligent civil servant had the inspiration that the Crown might be saved considerable expense if lepers could be cured by the waters of Kuppis instead of being sent to hospital. A proposal was therefore sent to the king in Stockholm, to which the following reply was received:

"To the Governor, Lorentz Creutz, a reply concerning the care of lepers in Åbo county.

Stockholm, April 16th, 1688

We have received your humble letter of March 31st from which we perceive that the infectious disease, leprosy, continues to increase in the country so that besides those in Själö hospital, a number of lepers in the early stages of the disease are to be found in Töfsala and in other parishes. It seems justified to try to treat those who this summer, as in previous years, will be taken to the hospital on the advice of Dr. Tillandz, who is too busy to treat them at the hospital which is three miles south of Åbo. We therefore graciously approve your humble proposal that a house should immediately be built in Åbo, where those who are in the early stages of this infectious disease should undergo a period of medical treatment, so that those who are potentially curable may not perish completely with the incurable, nor should they receive free food until their dying day if they can be made healthy and the hospital spared expense.

Carolus." (12)

Several buildings, including a sauna, were erected for the lepers that year in an area fenced off by Kuppis well. A "Kuppis watchman" was appointed and assigned an annual salary, which in the budget for the hospital in 1695 amounted to three tuns of corn. The buildings did not last long for they were burnt during hostilities between Sweden and Russia in 1713 and were not rebuilt. An annual blood-letting was suggested by the warden as an alternative treatment in 1731, and this the district surgeon professed himself "willing to do if he received something for his services". Nothing came of this suggestion, and no great imagination is needed to explain why.

Although the hospital authorities may have lost interest in the water of Kuppis well, the doctors at Åbo did not. In 1729, H. Spöring, then professor of medicine at Åbo, described the beneficial effect of Kuppis water in the case of Andrae Rusticus Wirmaensis, a leper who "in anxious quest for a cure of this malady ... soon sensibly went to a spring which owes its name to St. Henry, and which is otherwise known as Kuppis". First he bathed himself in the waters and later he started cautiously to imbibe, eventually taking "two whole pots and what overflowed" daily for a whole month, apparently with remarkable improvement in his condition. He was not, however, completely cured because the professor urged him to return for further treatment the following spring.

Not until the time of Welhaven in Bergen, in the early nineteenth century, is local treatment to prevent the worst mutilations of the disease described. These result from minor injuries to anaesthetic fingers and toes which become infected and eventually gangrenous. Welhaven was profoundly unimpressed with the result of all existing treatments, including the "rather expensive medicine" which he once procured from Dr. Monrad of Bergen and which he suspected had caused the "frenzy" in which the patient died. To Welhaven, the greatest challenge was to prevent gangrene in deformed fingers and toes. He once recalled "with a shudder that in my first year of office some died there of deep sores on their feet, which developed into gangrene for want of necessary care and medical assistance". Week by week, he procured from one of the city's apothecaries a variety of "salves, oils, salts, spices, and plaster". A salve was prepared and applied to their sores on absorbent paper. The patients mentioned that "without this salve, which cleans and soothes the sores, they could not bear the pain". Juniper oil was one of many remedies he purchased for them out of gifts to the hospital. Conventional measures of leeches, cupping, and bleeding were also employed as need arose, but without medical supervision.

The fact that no doctor attended the institution served only to impress upon the lepers that doctors had nothing to offer them. Welhaven summarised the situation thus:

> "The disease of these unfortunate people has been considered incurable, which the whole experience of the institution and its hospital is seen to prove, since no arrangements are made either for a doctor or for medicines for them." (13)

He did what he could to lighten their gloom and to relieve their suffering by making full use of gifts given to the hospital:

> "... through these gifts I have been enabled not only to procure medicaments and food, but also refreshments of tea, sugar, beer, and other dry and sweet refreshing drinks, indeed sometimes wine for the refreshment of the most sick; furthermore I sometimes obtained lint and linen for their many sores, of which they also have great need." (14)

But he failed to obtain the services of a doctor for them. Twenty years later there was still no doctor. The leper Peder Feidie (15) ruefully observed that people with other diseases in general hospitals fared much better:

"For other diseases found here
Wise doctors on the scene appear
Who understand disease.
To hospital those sick are brought
And for their plight a cure is sought;
Thus their ills are relieved,
And all their wounds are dressed

We lepers here can no doctors get:
Here must we stay and wait and fret
Until our time is up.
Peter from prison did escape
Because on God's grace he did wait;
O God, break now the chains
Which bind our limbs with pains."

The leper was under an immutable sentence of death, but execution was often more cruelly delayed than any legal sentence. His was a hopeless, helpless anguish, which made men and women hide their disease and carry on undetected for as long as possible. Pastor Muur was well acquainted with the problem amongst his people

> "... sometimes the housewife is a leper and has the house full of small children; rarely would she be willing to be parted from her children for a period of observation, indeed they would rather bear their burden and struggle on to the bitter end." (16)

The frustration and sorrow of broken lives, nostalgic memories, and unfulfilled hopes were ever-present companions. Peder Feidie described his own experience:

> "I was not yet 15 years old
> My mind was full of joys untold,
> Then were they all cut short.
> Pain overcame me and did start
> Quickly to pierce marrow, bone and heart.
> Oh, it was hard to bear
> This burden laid on me.
>
> Then for my father God did send,
> His misery now was at an end,
> His days on earth were done.
> Four children stood around the grave
> And watched with silent faces brave
> As his tired bones were laid
> In their earthy resting place."

Peder's eager, youthful expectations lay in ruins at his feet; like "captive Cresseid, now and ever more gone is your joy and all your happiness". To bear his own sorrows was hard enough, but he must also constantly endure the sufferings of his fellows.

> "Sometimes I softly walk about
> The silent house at evening time:
> Sorrowful sounds I hear.
> One bitterly cries 'woe is me',
> Another sighs and groans that he
> Must creep away to bed.
> Tell me O God—How long?"

"How long?"—we now know the answer to his plaintive question; it was seventeen long years before death finally released him from his suffering.

For some, the long years of a living death proved too much for their troubled conscience, as Welhaven once graphically recounted.

> "In the case of this woman, who died in the greatest misery, on whose body hardly a spot was free of sores, whose flesh was almost eaten away from fingers and toes, whose tongue and neck were seeded with boils, I made this strange discovery. One morning, when I came as priest to this sick woman's bedside I found her weeping. At once I enquired after the reason for her grief, which in any case I found understandable merely at the sight of that tormented person. But how great was my surprise when she said (referring to her husband who

had died from the same disease some time before) 'he was my brother. We were seven brothers and sisters', she continued, 'and that most leprous man was the youngest of us, and the six older were all free of the disease.'

"Astonished I asked after the condition of her parents and her other relations. 'Our parents', she continued, 'were healthy and only far back in our family did we know for certain that our father's aunt was just as severely leprous as this my wretched brother.'" (17)

Remarkably, many triumphed over their suffering and despair. The doctor who accompanied a French scientific expedition to Iceland in 1836 was shattered by the composure of an old woman, whom he described as the most horrible leper they saw on the island (Plate 35). "This woman", wrote Robert, "in spite of the horrible condition into which leprosy has cast her, and which she had suffered for two decades, did not seem overcome by sorrow, but was singing while M. Bevalet drew her portrait." Welhaven too remarked at the amazing fortitude of his flock; he described one young woman, the lower part of whose foot "hangs on by only a few sinews", who nevertheless was, "as are all the wretched company of lepers, extremely long-suffering in her severe torment".

Heaven was the leper's last and only hope. The medieval church had assured him that his sufferings would be rewarded there. The regulations of St. Julian's exhorted him to suffer his fate patiently—

"Nor should they despair or murmur against God ... but rather praise and glorify him who, when he was led to his death, wished to be compared to the lepers."

In the ordinances of their institution the lepers of Enköping were assured that they were "Yet heirs of God and co-heirs of Christ", and the service at the seclusion of a leper promised that "He may have a sure and certain hope that, though he be sick in body, he may be whole in soul and may obtain the gift of everlasting salvation." And de Chauliac had advised physicians to tell lepers that

"... the said disease is penance salutary for the salvation of their souls, and ... should be their purgatory in this world. For albeit they were refused of the world, yet they were and be chosen of God." (18)

Nothing had happened by the early nineteenth century to shake the medieval belief of men and women that they must bear their sufferings patiently for the present glory of God and for the eternal preservation of their own souls. Peder Feidie's verses could as well have been written in the twelfth century as in the nineteenth. His verses catch the atmosphere of seven centuries of desperate heavenly hope:

"In St. George's hospital here,
Sufferings over a hundred bear,
And wait to be set free.
O holy Ghost our helmsman true,
Steer us all our sufferings through
And to heaven lead us,
For there are we set free.

But even if our health be lost,
Yet are we not from God's sight tossed—

That can we daily see:
Wonderful gifts to us God sends
Provides us with kind unknown friends;
Both rich and poor are they
O Lord, do them repay.

Just so that everyone can see
That God cares for us tenderly,
Thus are we sorely scourged.
He gives and takes just as he will,
So take Lord from us our poor souls;
When from here we wander
Bring us to heaven's shore.

So now I end my humble song,
O God let not the time be long—
Thy will be done O Lord.
My wish it is, I who am weak,
After my death Thy throne to seek—
To praise thee and behold
Thy countless joys untold."

Heaven indeed offered the only hope: "with the doctors' best intention, insight, and industry", stated Welhaven at the same hospital a few years earlier, "it is impossible to heal the living dead".

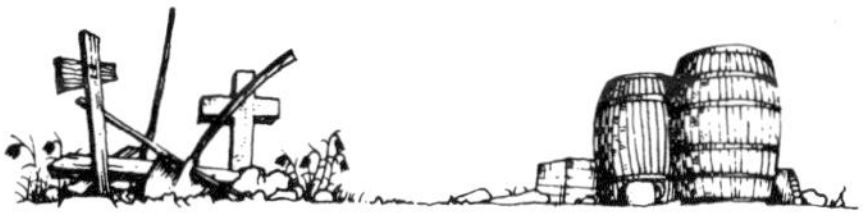

THE DISEASE

IX

The Rise and Fall of the Disease

Leprosy was becoming rare before leper hospitals declined. In the first half of the fourteenth century many hospitals already housed fewer lepers than their endowments could support. The Black Death may then have accelerated the decline of the disease, both by killing lepers and by reducing the total population. The latter effect was probably more important: premature death of lepers in hospital would have had an insignificant impact upon a disease more likely to be spread by unrecognised cases than by those sufficiently disfigured to be put away.

Lepers were no more and no less likely to have died from plague during the Black Death than inhabitants of equally humble dwellings. Plague, a disease of the house-rat which burrowed and nested in mud walls, floors, and in thatched roofs, reached man through the bite of rat fleas. Most leper hospitals were situated on the edge of towns, but this degree of isolation did not protect domestic rats from infection. Although lepers were not especially at risk from infection by plague, they were very vulnerable to its economic consequences. Dependent upon rents and charity for their survival, they were likely to be the first to starve in the economic dislocation which followed in the wake of the Black Death.

Many isolated regions escaped plague altogether. There, both life and leprosy continued their evolution without serious interruption. This may have been the most important reason why leprosy outlived the Middle Ages in the North, but it is unlikely to have been the only one.

By the fifteenth century the rarity of lepers is even more impressive than the dereliction of their hospitals. At Sherburn, in 1434, the establishment of 65 lepers and many priests was drastically reduced to a master, four chaplains, four clerks, two boys, thirteen poor men, one honest matron and two lepers, but the inclusion of paupers shows that even the reduced resources of the hospital were more than sufficient to support the available lepers. By 1552 Sherburn housed no lepers. Ripon leper hospital at the same period contained only two priests and five poor people to pray for all "Christen sowlez", while Ilford hospital, founded for thirteen lepers, two priests and a clerk could boast no more than "one pryest and two pore men". Shrewsbury hospital had been so long without lepers that the town had forgotten the purpose of its foundation: it was reported in the reign of King Henry VIII that the hospital had been "founded by the King's most noble progenitors, to what intent or purpose they cannot tell".

Only four new leper hospitals were founded in England in the sixteenth century—one in East Anglia, the others in Hereford, Dorset, and Devon. A few small pockets of infection probably survived into the early years of the next century in Devon and Cornwall. Scotland did not throw off leprosy so easily, indeed a new hospital was opened at the end of the sixteenth century, although it only accommodated a handful of lepers. Only in the Shetland islands is it reasonably certain that Scottish leprosy persisted into the eighteenth century.

Leprosy had become so rare in Denmark by the mid-sixteenth century that a law of 1542 transferred leper hospitals to the administration of local general hospitals for their use. The disease was probably equally rare in the south of Sweden, while in the north of Sweden and in Norway it continued at a low ebb. In Finland the situation was very different, for there the seventeenth century saw the peak of leprosy. Apart from the ill-fated hospital at Gloskär on the Åland islands, all the Finnish leper hospitals at this period differed from the traditional pattern, being built alongside an institution for the indigent and elderly infirm or, in the case of Själö hospital built on an island near Åbo in 1622, alongside a mad-house, part of which still exists. Själö hospital achieved a certain notoriety soon after its foundation when its first chaplain, Hieronymus Laurentii Hinnulinus, (no longer in the post at the time) was condemned to death for committing adultery. The two sections of these hospitals, often referred to as the "clean" and the "infectious" parts respectively, were under the same administration, but they strictly kept their own company with a few exceptions in the course of duty, such as a

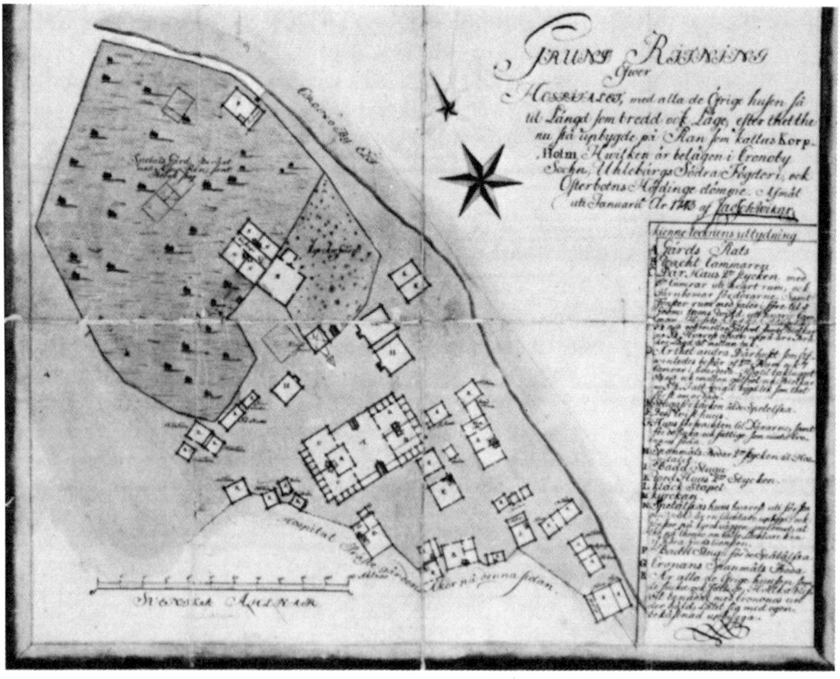

Plate 20. Ground plan of Kronoby hospital, Finland, in 1743. The hospital admitted both lepers and the elderly infirm. A stockade confined the lepers to the northern part of the site.

"clean" old man in Viborg hospital, who received an extra rye allowance for breaking the ice on the lepers' water supply in the winter.

The ground plan of Kronoby hospital in Finland (Plate 20), founded in 1631, shows clearly the separation of the lepers, whose area was sealed off by a stockade. There were only two gates in this fence, one of which led to their sauna on the

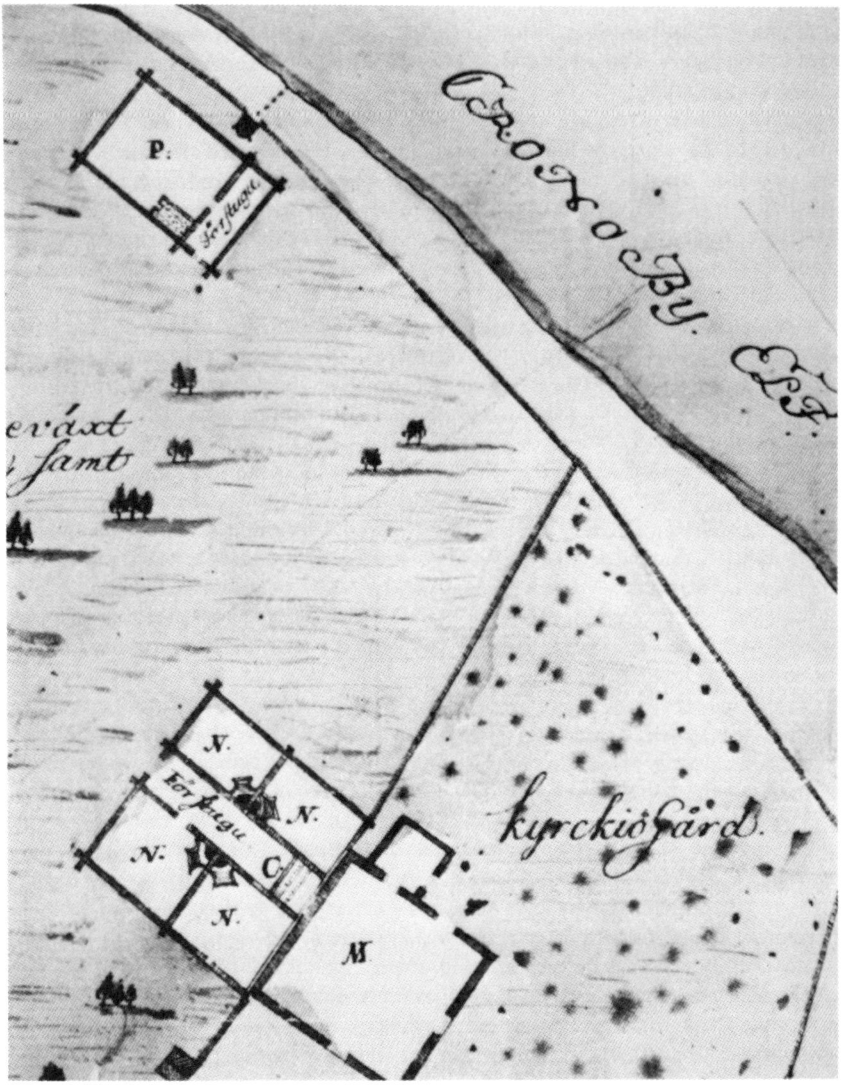

Plate 21. Detail of part of the ground plan of Kronoby hospital to show the lepers' dwellings (N) built against the north wall of the church (M) and the platform between them (O) from which the lepers could see through a window into the church and hear the service. A gate in the stockade gave them access to the river from their sauna (P).

river bank. They did not even have access to the church, against which their dwellings were built (Plate 21); they could only look through a window into the church by standing on a platform, perhaps the only authenticated leper window in history. It is uncertain whether the small windows found near the altar in many medieval churches really were leper "squints" as traditionally accepted, or whether they were confessionaries. The lepers at both Viborg and Själö attended the hospital chapel but sat in their own part of the church. At Viborg a railing separated the lepers from their "clean" brethren, while at Själö a screen walled off the south-west aisle used by the lepers; a small altar placed by an aperture in the screen enabled them to take communion.

A steady trickle of lepers entered the Finnish hospitals until the Russian occupation of 1713-22, when the lepers scattered. Few were admitted after the war; most had probably died of starvation. The last leper was admitted to Själö in 1766 and died in 1785. Kronoby hospital survived the war without damage, but in 1792 the lepers' quarters had been empty for so long that they were taken over for the use of mad patients. Thirty years later, however, it again became necessary to build accommodation for lepers.

Meanwhile, in Norway and Sweden a steady undercurrent of leprosy continued during the eighteenth century. Nevertheless, the disease was sufficiently uncommon in Sweden for Anton Martin, a Finnish medical student at Uppsala university, to visit Norway to study leprosy in 1759-60. There were then two leper hospitals in Norway: St. George's in Bergen, which had been rebuilt in 1702, and Reknæs hospital near Molde. It was rumoured at the time that leprosy was also a disease of fish and cattle: what better research project for a student in the age of Linnaeus than to examine this theory? Finding a leprous cow proved more difficult than expected, but in September, 1760, Martin heard of one and hastened to the scene. Alas, the carcass had already been buried officiously by a policeman. With laudable enterprise Martin records that "with pleading and payment I had it dug up again", and he performed a post-mortem examination on the spot.

The isolation of leper hospitals presented an unworthy opportunity which was not missed. Authority has been troubled throughout history by men close enough to the law to avoid prison, too sane for a mad-house, yet sufficiently discomforting to be put out of the way. Prominent amongst these in Sweden and Finland in the eighteenth century were dissenting pietists, several of whom ended their days in the "clean" section of leper hospitals in Finland. One such, Olaf Norman, caused great consternation in Sweden in the 1730s and was declared to be incorrigible by Bishop Rydelius, who personally attempted to dissuade him from his heretical views. For a time Norman was confined in Kalmar castle in southern Sweden, but even here he succeeded in obtaining sufficient freedom to gain more adherents. His views were considered so dangerous that, in 1741, the bishop proposed that this otherwise mild and inoffensive man should be transported to a suitably remote place in Finland near the Russian frontier; he went so far as to envisage a remote separatist colony supporting itself by its own labours in an environment where, surrounded by neighbours of Orthodox religion, there was no danger of the spread of irreligious doctrines (at least, not to good Lutherans).

Eventually Norman and his family were transported to Finland to be put away in Själö hospital. They wintered in Åbo castle because no house had yet been built for them on the hospital site. On May 11th, 1745, when the sea-ice had broken up, they were taken by boat to the island of Själö, but not before Norman had deeply influenced the chaplain of Åbo castle with his views. Even at Själö, Norman remained a thorn in the flesh of the authorities; not least in 1751, when, on the death of one of his children, he buried the child in his kitchen garden in accordance with his dissenting doctrine, an action which the authorities condemned as highly reprehensible "self-indulgence". Norman lived in remote isolation in the company of madmen, and a stone's throw from the lepers, until his death in 1773 at the age of 85 (1).

Throughout Finland and the north of Sweden, around the eastern shores of the Baltic, and particularly on the west coast of Norway, leprosy increased steadily early in the nineteenth century, in some places to an alarming extent. In 1836, a petition was put before the Norwegian parliament requesting more hospitals for lepers: a Royal Commission was appointed and one new hospital, Lungegårds hospital, was opened in Bergen in 1849. Twenty years later, a census of lepers counted an astonishing total of 2,858 in a population of 1,500,000—a modest enough incidence (2 per 1,000) over the whole country, but leprosy was almost entirely confined to the west coast; here, in the worst affected communities, twenty to twenty-five people in every 1,000 were suffering from leprosy. Something had to be done.

Two new leper hospitals were built and two existing hospitals were enlarged. New leper hospitals were built at Bergen (Pleistiftelse no. 1, curiously named when it was the third leper hospital in the city), and at Reknæs near Molde, on the coast between Bergen and Trondheim. The old St. George's hospital at Bergen and the hospital for lepers at Trondheim were enlarged.

From that moment leprosy declined. Observers claimed this as a triumph for isolation, even the Prince of Wales, who visited Trondheim leper hospital in 1885, referred to Norway as a "shining example of a land where they grieve for the misery of lepers and where great results have been obtained" (2). The truth is different. At no time were more than one third of the lepers in Norway in hospital (Plate 22), and even they were not strictly isolated. A visitor to Norway in 1889 recorded that

> "The isolation of lepers is not absolute. The doors and gates of the institutions are not locked, and more than once I met some of the inmates on the neighbouring roads. ... The lepers are, however, usually kept in on market days and, at Trondheim at least and I believe elsewhere, they are not permitted to enter houses or churches, or to come into close contact with other people." (3)

As so often happens, the crisis was over before action was taken. Leprosy had already passed its peak in Norway by 1856. In spite of more than one thousand new cases in the next decade (Plate 23), the total number of lepers in the country fell steadily (Plate 22). Such was the rapidity of the decline that in 1895 Lungegårds hospital in Bergen was converted into a school and Reknæs hospital near Molde became a tuberculosis sanitorium. In 1925, the Trondheim leper hospital was converted into a lunatic asylum, and the following year the demise of the seven remaining patients in St. George's hospital in Bergen was awaited by the authorities who planned "to demolish the old building and to avail themselves of its ample and well-situated site in the centre of the town". In fact it still stands (Plate 7). After the second world war only Pleistiftelse no. 1 remained in use: in 1957 it housed just four leprosy patients and was closed soon afterwards.

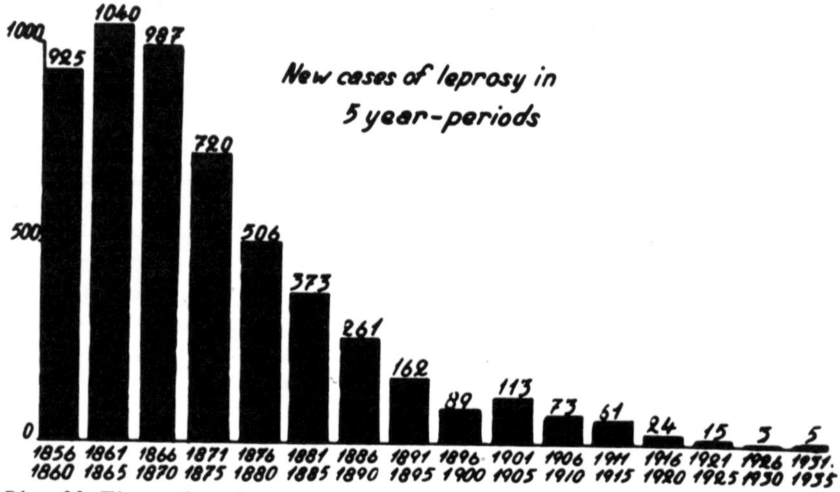

Plate 22. The number of new cases of leprosy reported in Norway from 1856 to 1935.

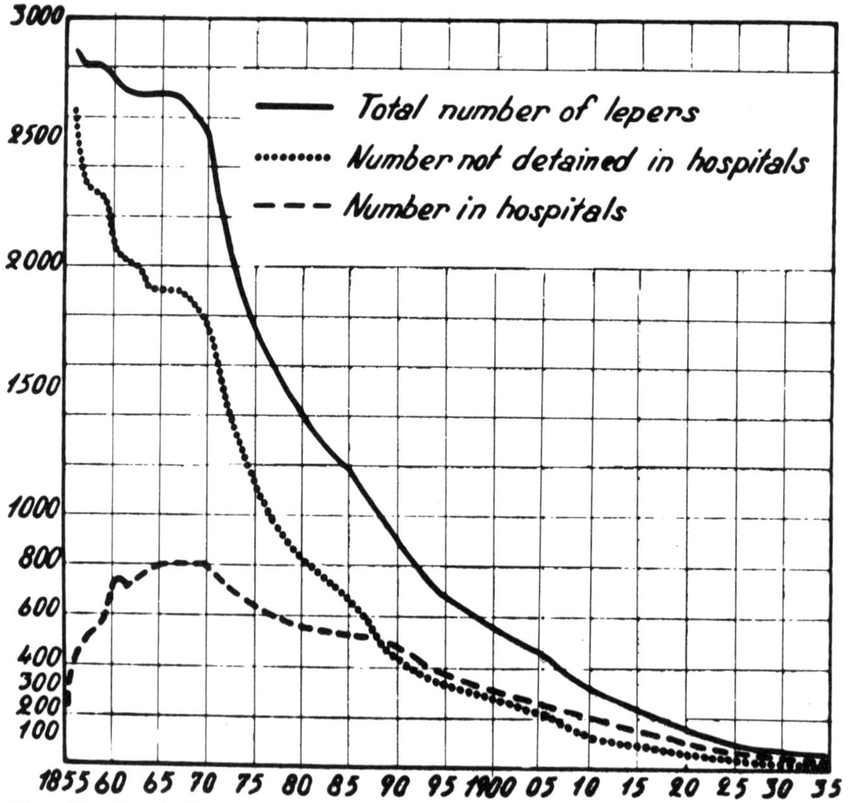

Plate 23. Graph showing the total number of lepers in Norway from 1856 to 1935 and the number of those isolated in hospital. During the most rapid decline of the disease no more than one third of the lepers were in hospital.

Although past its peak before a census was taken, leprosy had achieved such momentum in Norway that a total of 8,224 cases were reported between 1856 and 1956. The last three cases were diagnosed in 1951, a man and his two sisters who had never left the country but who had had two leprous aunts many years previously. Only today is it at last certain that this long chapter in Norwegian history is finally closed.

Leprosy continued to be a problem in several Swedish counties north of Stockholm into this century. Parish records in the county of Hälsingland from 1810 to 1856 gave leprosy (in its local name of *Knölsjuka*—"lump disease") as the cause of death of 97 people. Following the Norwegian example, a hospital was founded at Järvsö in 1864, and it was extended several times. Between 1861 and 1908 more than 600 cases of leprosy were notified in Sweden, and even between 1923 and 1937 a further 17 cases were reported. The continuity of the disease in some parishes was most impressive. In the mid-eighteenth century the parish of Älvkarleby in the county of Uppland was such a focus of leprosy that the disease became widely known as "Älvkarleby-disease" (4). Between 1883 and 1892, more than a century after it acquired this name, seven of the 106 new cases of leprosy in Sweden were from that same parish of Älvkarleby. By 1955, only three leprosy patients remained in Sweden: two had never been out of the country and the third was an Estonian who had entered the country in 1944. The Baltic states of Estonia, Latvia, and Lithuania have a long history of leprosy (5). Baltic Russia was not spared either: 49 cases of leprosy were treated in St. Petersburg between 1877 and 1889, half of whom came from the city itself (6).

The highest number of lepers recorded in Finland in the last hundred years was 95 in 1904, the year that an old army barracks at Orivesi was converted into a leper hospital. Orivesi hospital closed in 1953 when its remaining three patients were transferred to a hospital near Helsingfors, where their two major consolations were a framed letter of 1930 from President Relander of Finland promising them that "behind dark clouds the wonderful clear sun is shining" (7), and a conducted tour of Helsingfors by car twice a year to remind them of the world outside. Three other patients were at home in different parts of the country. Of the four in hospital in 1956 none had ever travelled abroad and two had no idea of any possible source of infection; the other two had leprous relatives, but one of them had never even met the relative in question. The last case of leprosy in Finland was diagnosed in 1955.

In Iceland, Scandinavian in both blood and traditions, the last case was diagnosed in 1956, a 60-year-old woman who from the age of 6 to 18 had lived with an aunt who subsequently developed leprosy (8). The highest number of cases in Iceland, as in Norway, was recorded at the time of the first extensive (but not exhaustive) search for the disease. Although probably well past its peak, 236 cases were identified in 1896 in a population of 75,000, an incidence of three per 1,000—greater even than in Norway. Most cases were in south-western coastal districts. The following year a leper hospital was opened at Laugarnes near Reykjavik. By 1910, only 96 lepers were known, and in 1957 there were only 8. About 10,000 cases of leprosy were recorded in Norway, Sweden, Finland, and Iceland between 1856 and 1956.

Ideas about the nature of leprosy changed very little until the end of the nineteenth century. By the seventeenth century these ideas had polarised into two conflicting opinions: one, which might be called the Atlantic view, represented the majority opinion in Norway, Iceland, and the Faroes that leprosy was not infectious; the other, the Baltic view, is typified by the attitude seen in Finland and current also in Sweden, which arose directly out of the late medieval fear of infection.

The Atlantic view was taking shape on the Faroe islands in 1676. At this time, as Pastor Derbes recorded, they accepted that the disease might be spread by contact and, like the people of Åland, suspected that the incubation period might be very long; nevertheless they noted that even those in close contact for many years frequently did not acquire the disease. They did not consider the risk of catching the disease sufficiently great to rule their lives:

> "... the disease acting a great while in a man before it breaketh out, it happeneth that many think they be clean on both sides do marry together and yet afterwards the one is found to be infected. God and nature deal wonderfully with such people in their marriage, for amongst the children they beget, some are clean and some are unclean ... wherefore the inhabitants take but little care in their wooing whether the parents have been clean or no.
>
> It has been noted that two living together in marriage, though the one be found infected... yet the second remaineth unaffected; whereas another is often taken by the disease by a very little conversation. ... What is this but that God confirms the truth of his word, taking pleasure in them that live in a just wedlock and wander in lawful ways. ..." (9)

A century later in Norway, neither the two parish priests, Møller and Strøm, who described the disease in their parishioners, nor the medical student Anton Martin during his year in Bergen, indicate that people feared that lepers would infect them. Certainly centuries earlier, in 1325, Bishop Håkon had confirmed an ancient law forbidding lepers to live amongst other folk in order to prevent the spread of the disease, but there is no suggestion that the purpose of eighteenth-century Norwegian leper hospitals was to remove sources of infection from society, indeed the opposite is true. Martin states that the hospitals for lepers opened by the State at Trondheim, Molde and Bergen were to look after "such unfortunate people until the day of their death". The same was true of Iceland, where Petersen comments that the five hospitals for lepers were opened "for the poorest of them, not with a view to treatment but rather so that they could have food and shelter". Indeed he was aware that if treatment were possible the problem would be greater, because the longer the lepers survived in hospital the fewer the number who could be offered shelter "because the hospital's money is insufficient for many to be sustained at once".

In Norway and Iceland in the early nineteenth century neither priests, doctors, nor people feared infection by leprosy. Not only were relatives of patients allowed to visit St. George's hospital in Bergen, but Welhaven records that they had "eaten with them out of the same dish, slept in their beds immediately after they had got up and the bed was still warm, without the least harmful consequence for their health". Also local people attended services in the hospital chapel, pushed their way into the same pews as the patients and "in the extreme summer heat pack themselves tight together even with the most ill of them, without the least fear". So insignificant was any thought of acquiring leprosy to the women who acted as nurses in the hospital that they sometimes retired there and lived "under the same conditions as the Institution's other sick members". Thorsteinsson, an Icelandic physician of the same period, stated categorically that "leprosy is not regarded on Iceland to be infectious, but is hereditary here".

Paradoxically, the more penetratingly critical the observation of the disease the more difficult it became to accept that it was infectious. This now makes sense because it has been established that individual susceptibility varies greatly, and the incubation period may extend over decades. But to Welhaven, chaplain to St. George's hospital in Bergen for the first quarter of the nineteenth century, and to the Norwegian doctors D. C. Danielssen and C. W. Boeck, who in 1847 published the first scientific monograph on leprosy, the gulf between the theory of infection and their own observations was too wide to span. Welhaven's analysis was a triumph of observation and critical reasoning, untutored by any medical training, and perhaps all the better for that. He considered one by one the many current theories of the causation of the disease only to end unconvinced and baffled; in his view the theories were "only guesses ... plausible to a point" but no further.

No theory satisfactorily explained all the facts before him. How should he interpret a situation in which the first three children of a healthy woman with a "healthy and dexterous husband" all developed leprosy and died, wheareas the fourth child born after the mother had at last developed signs of leprosy herself "still lives at home in the parish, is 42 years old, and is a farm-worker with good and strong health"? Lepers commonly had leprous relatives but Welhaven could point to many healthy children of leprous parents. Petter Olofsson (Plate 24), who was

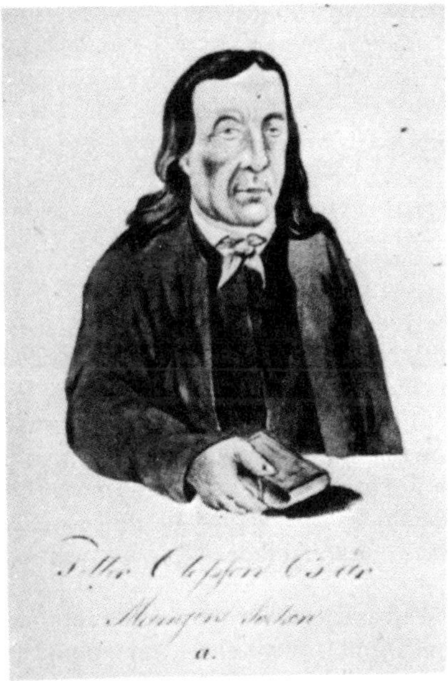

Plate 24. Petter Olofsson.

in the hospital as Welhaven wrote, had been suspected to have leprosy when his leprous mother brought him with her to the hospital when he was 9 years old. Either the diagnosis was incorrect or, as rarely happens, he had recovered spontaneously, for when Welhaven sketched him after fifty-four years in the hospital he showed no signs of leprosy.

Could a man have escaped both his mother's disease and the disease of those all around him for half a century if it really were infectious? Welhaven recalled that throughout all those years Olofsson had slept in a little overcrowded dormitory with highly leprous people, eaten and drunk out of the same vessel, and lived in close contact with the other patients, "yet, one cannot detect the least sign of leprosy on the whole of his body, on the contrary he enjoys excellent health and has especially good strength". Another man, Hindrick Ottosson (Plate 25), who

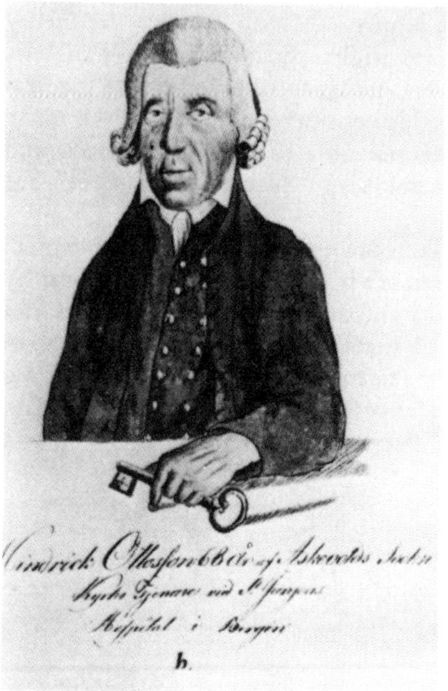

Plate 25. Hindrick Ottoson.

at the age of 68 was celebrating his fiftieth year in the hospital, was equally remarkable. His parents were healthy, and it will never be known whether he really had leprosy when admitted to the hospital at the age of 18. The fact remains that he had endured constant "close and daily contact with the patients" and now had no evidence of the disease. Both these men could probably have left the hospital years ago, like a young woman who, after observation in the hospital for some years, was permitted to go into service in the town. But they had lost touch with the outside world, and now had no alternative but to stay on in spite of the miserable conditions and horrifying company. Ottosson became verger to the hospital chapel. Olofsson appears from his portrait to have learned to read, but his function in the hospital is not recorded.

The "graveyard of the living" over which Welhaven presided was a tidy solution to the problem posed by those who could not support themselves and whom the community preferred to be without; it did not exist because of a threat to the health of others. Unlike Erik of Norboda on Åland who was forbidden to sell the gloves he made because of the danger that they might transmit his infection, the lepers of Bergen were encouraged to occupy their time gainfully. The women spun flax, tow hemp and wool, sewed, knitted, and wove. The men made sea-boots, shoes, ladles, vats, tubs, agricultural implements, and fishing nets.

Against this background of disbelief that leprosy was infectious, it would be a mistake to see the demand of 1836 for more leper hospitals in Norway, or the expansion of hospitals twenty years later, as attempts to prevent the spread of the disease. Not until several years after the discovery of the leprosy bacillus by G. A. Hansen in 1873 did medical opinion in Norway (and Norway was second to none in the nineteenth century as an opinion on leprosy) swing towards infection from person to person as the mode of transmission of the disease. Now it seems obvious, then it was not. Neither Danielssen nor Boeck, founders of the scientific study of leprosy and Hansen's senior colleagues in Bergen, could accept that the bacillus discovered by Hansen in leprous nodules was the cause of the disease, nor that it proved that it was infectious. Only the bacteria causing anthrax had already been described, and the tuberculosis bacillus, the next to be discovered, was not announced until nine years later. Acceptance of the leprosy bacillus as the cause of the disease was further delayed because, unlike other bacteria causing disease, it could not be cultured outside the body, nor could it be shown to cause the disease when inoculated into another individual.

In spite of medical equivocation the Norwegian parliament cautiously passed a law in 1877 that lepers must either enter hospital or be isolated at home. A stricter law followed in 1885, which authorised the forcible removal to hospital of those who did not comply with the rules of home isolation, a law which was repealed as recently as January 1st, 1965. Lepers were not forbidden to marry in Norway (a bill to that effect had been rejected in 1845), but in 1918 a law was passed which permitted a leper to marry only if the healthy partner was aware of the disease and if both partners had been advised by a doctor concerning the potential danger of infection; this law lasted until 1969.

Iceland was only slowly converted to the Atlantic view of the disease. Besides being the only country to prohibit the marriage of lepers by law (in 1776), they still in the eighteenth century used to mutter "He is a leper: may God be near us and watch over us" when they saw a leper, a reaction which implies fear of infection, although it might be argued that it only displays concern for self-preservation whatever the unknown cause of the disease. On the other hand, they did not pretend that the purpose of isolation in hospital was anything other than humanitarian. In 1898, Icelanders still acknowledged the possibility of infection but were not overwhelmed by it; a law of that year (10) decreed that married couples should not be separated against their will unless a doctor considered that "the disease or danger of infection is of such a serious character that removal to hospital is necessary". Married couples were the one exception to the rule contained in that law that "lepers must not share a bed with others", a reminder of the days when the household and even visitors shared the one bed. Whatever the law said, however, the people displayed singularly little fear of infection.

The Danish leprosy-specialist Ehlers recorded an incident during his medical survey in 1895 when a 34-year-old woman with advanced leprosy

> "... came to me on horseback accompanied by a dead-drunk attendant. Need I add that they both employed the same pocket flask of brandy, regardless of the large ulcerated lepromata in the woman's throat, on her lips, and on her tongue." (11)

He was also told that four years earlier a child on a farm had shared the bed of a leper for a year and a half. The most macabre bed-sharing was the case of a woman in labour whose doctor had visited the house only the day before to certify the death of a leper. To his horror

> "The woman in labour lay in the same bed with the same bedclothes which the leprous corpse had left the day before ... the same winter the woman in labour was attacked by tuberous leprosy." (12)

Paradoxically, at the very moment that the Atlantic school was being persuaded that leprosy was in fact infectious, the Baltic school, which had been convinced since the Middle Ages that it was both infectious and dangerous, changed its mind. During the eighteenth century it had remained true to its traditional view, and in 1765 a young Finnish doctor, Isaac Uddman, stated clearly in the first M.D. thesis on leprosy that the purpose of leper hospitals in Finland was to prevent lepers "infecting" others. But in 1875, while Norway was insisting on the isolation of lepers at home or in hospital, Finland passed a law excluding incurable patients (and lepers were still incurable) from hospital; the one exception was made that a few lepers could be admitted to a separate part of the university of Helsingfors hospital for diseases of the skin and venereal disease "where they could serve to the instruction of young doctors". Both Finland and Sweden weathered the nineteenth-century explosion of leprosy without laws to force lepers to hospital; only public opinion forced those who absconded from hospital to return. Since 1945, Finnish lepers have been obliged to accept treatment at home or in hospital.

A second and more explicable paradox is the fact that the Shetland Isles were Baltic not Atlantic in their philosophy towards leprosy. Undoubtedly this was because their traditions in the eighteenth century were firmly medieval Scottish. No ambiguity surrounds the measures taken on Shetland in the eighteenth century: prevention of infection, even infection carried on the wind, was their purpose. Andrew Fisken, minister of Delting, Walls, and Sandnes wrote in 1736 of lepers in his parish:

> "The persons that fall into this direful case are, as soon as it is observed, obliged to retire to a solitary little hut, built on purpose for them at a distance from all houses, and are not allowed any converse with their husbands, wives or nearest relations, but have their necessaries of life furnished them by a contribution from all the inhabitants of the isle, and brought to their hut, which they take in when the person who has brought it has retired to the windward of their house at some distance." (13)

A few years later a unique and momentous celebration was arranged. For the first time in living memory the island of Papa was free from the "infectious disease" of leprosy—or so they thought. The session records of the parish of Walls record that on March 17th, 1742,

> "The Moderator proposed to the Session that considering that a Gracious Providence had not only delivered the Island and Country from the burden and necessity of maintaining and otherwise providing for the poor Lepers formerly in their Island, but had also put a stop to the spreading of that unclean and infectious disease, so that there is no appearance of the symptoms thereof in any person now in this place, the Session should therefore ordain a day to be set apart for solemn thanksgiving for so great a deliverance throughout this ministry excepting Fowla, which we have no access properly to inform." (13)

Thus remote little Fowla missed the solemn day of thanksgiving celebrated on May 19th, 1742, held, one suspects, more out of canny relief at the lifting of a costly burden from the shoulders of the impecunious parishioners than out of deep gratitude to heaven for closing a very long chapter of human misery and distress. The thanksgiving proved premature for, in 1772, Margaret Abernethy was found to have leprosy, to the consternation of parents who "were in the greatest fear that their children would be infected by her".

Many theories have been advanced to explain the rise and fall of leprosy in Europe; most of these theories fit many of the facts, but none satisfactorily explains them all. The medieval hypothesis that leprosy was caused by excessive consumption of rotten fish was still current early in the twentieth century. It was seriously discussed (by an Englishman) at the second International Leprosy Conference, which was held at Bergen in 1909 as a tribute to Norwegian contributions to leprosy research. Both leprosy and the consumption of fish were noted to have declined at the time of the Reformation (the decline in leprosy had, as discussed, begun long before), except in coastal areas of Norway, Sweden, Finland, and Iceland where both the dietary habit and the disease continued. There is no evidence, however, that either the amount of fish eaten or its rottenness increased when leprosy made a strong recovery nearly three centuries later. Fish was supplemented by seal meat in coastal areas of Finland, the excessive consumption of which was also blamed for leprosy.

Medieval physicians had coupled fish and milk as causes of leprosy. A Danish physician, Engelbreth, was not impressed by the fish-story, but thought that the cause was in goat's milk. In a closely reasoned historical argument (14) he claimed that leprosy was a variety of goat tuberculosis. Goats became such a nuisance in Denmark that Christian III, the same king who had closed the leper hospitals in 1542, ordered that goats should only be kept on open moorland. Engelbreth believed that Christian III's two greatest (and closely inter-related) achievements were to rid Denmark of goats and of leprosy. He failed to mention that leprosy disappeared from England at about the same time without a crusade against goats. It was true, however, that goat's milk was, and still is, commonly used in Norway; on the other hand there was no evidence that goats were more tuberculous or that more of their milk was consumed in those parts of the country worst affected by leprosy. At least his theory took more account of the facts than the evergreen theory which has been invoked to explain almost every disaster throughout history: on this occasion it was a Norwegian, Bucholz, who declared that leprosy was "a direct result of a deep spiritual and moral stagnation, and the consequent physical degeneration". (15)

Leprosy thrives on poor living conditions and poor diet; close contact is normally necessary for its transmission. Living conditions certainly were primitive where the disease prospered, but evidence is lacking that conditions were worse in the early nineteenth century than immediately before or afterwards, or indeed that they were worse in areas affected by leprosy than in those which were not. It is also not proved, although it seems to be so, that poor nutrition increases susceptibility to leprosy. Towards the end of the century, when the disease was in rapid decline, conditions were still extremely bad. A traveller in western Norway in 1873 wrote:

"... the food is of the most miserable description. ... In agricultural matters the natives of the western districts are at least two centuries behind the rest of the world . . . not only is the quality of the food extremely bad, but the quantity is often insufficient; during a hard winter many deaths occur from starvation." (16)

On his visit to Iceland in 1895 Ehlers commented on the poor diet and described the living conditions thus:

> "The Icelandic habitation is in its typical form a sod-hut of green turf . . . The front is covered with a thin layer of boards, some few of the rooms are boarded and from the boards drips moisture in big drops, even in fine weather, for the sod absorbs dampness like a sponge. In the facade are some few windows which are all, however, nailed up for fear of the winter cold. . . . One of the rooms always serves as separate bedroom for the peasant and his wife; but with the poor this room is dropped and all the people of the farm—men, women and children—sleep in the same room, the so-called Badstofa. . . . If you enter this Badstofa when thirteen or fourteen persons lie sleeping there, first of all you feel a temperature which certainly, both summer and winter reminds you of the tepidarium of a Roman bath, but surely here the likeness ceases. A suffocating stink and an unwholesome smell meets you. . . . In this dirt a confused mixture of cats, dogs and children lie reeking on the floor exchanging caresses and parasites . . ." (17)

It is difficult to think of a disease which would not flourish under these conditions, yet at that moment leprosy was declining.

Judged from the failure of leprosy to establish itself amongst Scandinavian settlers who took the disease with them to the Mississippi valley, where for several decades they lived in conditions similar to those they had left at home (18), harsh conditions are not enough to perpetuate the disease. Approximately 175,000 Norwegians emigrated to North America in the second half of the nineteenth century, including 170 lepers, only 30 of whom were known to have the disease when they left Norway (19). Not only does leprosy need a substantial minimum number of lepers in a community to survive, but the susceptibility of the members of the community seems crucial.

The population was increasing in the early nineteenth century in spite of hard living conditions, and those families genetically most susceptible to infection probably increased in proportion. Intermarriage within families was common in isolated communities and susceptible families may in this way have become even more likely to develop the disease on slight infection. Certainly the disease had a striking familial incidence: in Iceland in 1837, for example, hardly any of the 125 registered lepers was without affected relations. A large number of people particularly at risk may have been enough by itself to give new impetus to the disease.

Why then, without improved economic conditions, and with the population increasing, did leprosy soon start to decline again? Isolation was neither sufficiently general nor strict enough to be a significant factor. Withdrawal of the old Norwegian right (*lagd*) to wander from farm to farm receiving hospitality in 1877 may have reduced the spread of the disease more effectively than the isolation of late and obvious cases in hospital, but again this measure was far too late to explain the decline. One of the most important factors may have been the parallel increase in tuberculosis. One in three lepers dying in Norwegian hospitals in the second half of the nineteenth century and one in five in Iceland in this century died of tuberculosis. But the part played by tuberculosis in the defeat of leprosy cannot be more than guessed at until more is known about the timing of the rise in tuberculosis itself. Also there is no reason to believe that tuberculosis was responsible for the medieval decline of leprosy. Drugs effective against leprosy have only been available for thirty years, too late to help more than the last handful of Scandinavian lepers, and far too late to make any contribution to the decline of the disease.

Neither the medieval ebbing of leprosy, nor its explosion in the nineteenth century, nor its extinction in the twentieth century can be completely explained by any single factor. Doubtless many circumstances have contributed to differing extents at different times. It is not even possible to be sure whether the bacillus itself waxed and waned in virulence or whether the resistance of the people to it altered. Only joint study of communities at different periods by medical epidemiologists, economic historians, and social historians can hope to explain the curious facts of the changing fortunes of this disease. Study of contemporary communities which escaped leprosy is just as important as examination of those seriously affected; without such comparison no conclusions can be drawn. Only one fact is certain: leprosy is now dead in the North for the first time since the Middle Ages.

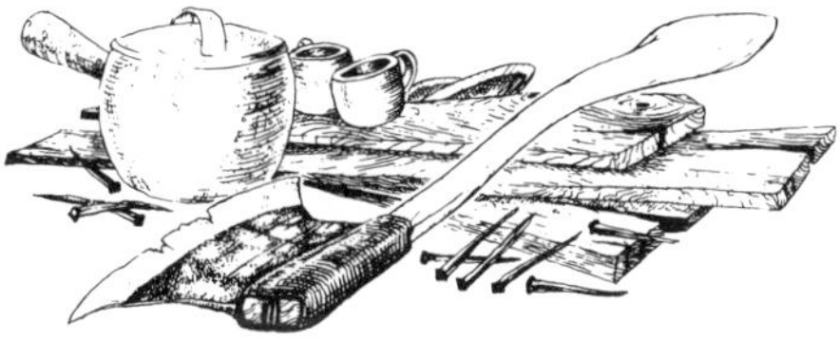

X

Leprosy—Fact or Fiction?

1. *An unbroken chain*

Medieval leprosy makes a fascinating tale—but is the story true? Was the disease really leprosy, or was the name given indiscriminately to many disfiguring diseases (as has often been said)? Its medical identity is not important to this pageant of attitudes, fears, and fate, except in that the reality of the disease provides a yardstick against which to measure one small fragment of history. If it could be shown that the tradition was indeed founded on the accurate recognition of one disease, then the rest of the story might be accepted not as folklore but fact.

Few doubt that medieval physicians recognised the most distinctive features of leprosy, but for many centuries doctors were not commonly involved in the diagnosis. Priests and people were the arbiters of the disease. The very fact that leprosy undoubtedly survived in Norway, Iceland, Finland, and Sweden until a few years ago strongly suggests that the same disease has continued since the Middle Ages, but was it correctly recognised? Descriptions, pictures, and the bones of the lepers themselves indicate that it was.

The standard fourteenth-century medical descriptions were clearly founded on personal experience. In both the *Lilium Medicinae* of Bernhard Gordon, professor of medicine at Montpelier, and the *Compendium Medicinae* of Gilbert Anglicus, leprosy was divided into three stages. The first signs were described as a repugnant appearance, a dusky redness of the face, harshness of the voice, thinning and falling of hair, and widespread scabs, boils, and nodules. In the second stage the eyebrows enlarged, the nostrils became swollen and obstructed, the voice sounded nasal, lumps, which frequently ulcerated, appeared on the ear lobes, face, and elsewhere, and symptoms of involvement of nerves were described, such as a 'pins-and-needles' sensation and wasting of muscles. Finally, the tissues of the nose were destroyed, breathing became difficult, the voice sounded rough and hoarse, the lips were thickened, the face looked horribly disfigured, and both the feet and hands became mutilated.

These books were read in England, and their descriptions were copied by John of Gaddesden a few years later at Merton College, Oxford. Later in the fourteenth century, another English work, *De Proprietatibus Rerum* by Bartholomew Glanville, gave a similar but possibly partly original account of the disease: he described the sufferers as "... unclene, spotyd, glemy and quyttery, the Nosethrills ben stopyl, the wasen of Voys is rough, the Voys is horse and the Heere falls".

The most influential of all the medieval descriptions of leprosy (*lepra arabum* or *elefantiasis*) was contained in *Inventarium sive Collectorium Partis Chirugicalis Medicinae* by Guy de Chauliac, first published in 1363. This book became a standard medical and surgical text in Western Europe. It not only promoted a precise and detailed medical examination of those suspected to have the disease, but introduced the idea that the degree of isolation to be enforced should depend on the certainty of diagnosis, which was to be judged from a number of "equivocal" and "unequivocal" signs. The unequivocal signs included thickening and tuberosity of the eyebrows with loss of their hair, disfiguration and obstruction of the nostrils, a harsh and nasal voice, scarring around the eyes and ears, and a horrible, satyr-like appearance.

These medieval criteria were still used on the Åland islands in the seventeenth century. At Sund on February 21st, 1648, Märta of Finneby was suspected of leprosy for two particular reasons: her voice had "changed considerably" and her skin "had altered to a bluish brown colour". She was put under observation at home for one year to await developments. Sometimes several years elapsed before a certain diagnosis could be made. For four and a half years Erik Jönsson of Notö laboured under suspicion of leprosy because of deformity and swelling of his face with a variable alteration in his voice, but Muur considered that "he cannot be proved for certain". The case of Erik of Norboda was reviewed many times. As early as 1646 the doctors in Stockholm were unsure, and it was reported that he "cannot obtain from the doctors a certificate of freedom from leprosy"; he was ordered to "live in an outhouse completely removed from society". At one time he seemed to be improving because his face was less swollen, his beard had grown again, his skin had considerably improved, and his voice was "almost normal". The parish still cautiously ordered him to remain under observation in his house. In 1650, the parish was instructed that he should again be "thoroughly inspected" one Sunday, "if he has the strength to walk to the church"; once again no diagnosis could be made. Their caution was eventually vindicated, for in January 1651 it was announced that "Erik of Norboda is a leper". Muur did not bother to record reasons for sure diagnosis, probably because they were too well-known to be repeated; only when there was doubt were the symptoms and signs recorded.

It was said of a woman called Kaisa in Föglö in 1648 that "her face has become worse, her body is diseased, but her voice is not too bad". In 1650, the sheriff's officer at Sund appointed men of the parish to examine the wife of a man called Cnut, telling them to check on "her skin, voice, and limbs, those parts of the body where leprosy is found". Limbs also figure in the case of "Kaarin of Hummelsöö" who was isolated at home on suspicion of leprosy. In 1640, she sent word to the parish of Föglö that her face had become darker and more swollen. One of the parishioners was sent to visit her, and reported back that "her head and feet remain diseased, but few faults were found with her voice". A similar view of the disease prevailed on the Faroe islands where Pastor Derbes wrote in 1676 that

> "The Leprosie wherewith they are troubled in this country is usually *Elephantiasis*, for the face and limbs of almost all the infected are full of blew knobs that break out sometimes as Boyles, whereby they look very deformed in the face, being besides all hoarse and speaking through their noses." (1)

Mutilations of hands and feet were rarely mentioned. Possibly they were too commonplace to report, but more likely few lepers lived long enough to get them. Mutilations were, however, reported in a young man admitted to Själö hospital in 1722. Leprosy had started ten years earlier when he was only 8 years old, but his admission to hospital had been prevented by the Russian occupation of

Finland. By the time he was finally admitted, all hope of recovery had been abandoned "because during the Russian rule no treatment could be obtained, and not only his face, but one hand and one foot are irretrievably spoilt". For this, at least, the Russians could not fairly be blamed; no effective treatment existed either before or after their invasion! It is likely that his long survival was in no small measure due to the fact that he could not go to hospital. Life was longer at home.

In 1738, at Åbo not far from Själö hospital, the professor of medicine, H. Spöring, published the first Scandinavian case report of leprosy:

> "Henricus Andrae Rusticus Wirmaensis was suffering from early signs of a severe form of leprosy: swellings of diverse size afflicted his entire body. ... At first dark, the swellings soon became reddish-blue (*livida*). ... His nostrils broke out into similar eruptions, so that he could only breathe through his mouth and then with difficulty. His voice was hoarse and whistling in character; the hairs on chin and eyebrows were sparse and falling out. ... All his skin was dry, rough, and shrivelled. ... The superficial swellings appeared particularly livid, becoming fissured and exuding sanguinous fluid. ... His feet were more swollen than the remainder of his body, and suffered rather slighter and flattish ulcerations associated with a sensation of numbness." (2)

His account unmistakably describes the same disease as this description written in 1974:

> "... a variety of lesions will be found on examination—macules, papules, and nodules. Macules ... with an erythematous or coppery sheen. ... The patient should be questioned about nasal symptoms such as blockage ... and also about oedema (swelling) of the legs and feet as these symptoms are common early manifestations of lepromatous leprosy ... the skin becomes thickened, the eyebrows become thinned or lost, the nose becomes broadened and deformed, the ear lobes are thickened, the voice becomes hoarse ... and a slow fibrosis takes place in peripheral nerves." (3)

Strikingly similar eye-witness accounts appeared over the next half century in Norway, Sweden, and Iceland—not as a new disease but as an old and familiar one, which for one reason or another was attracting new interest. It may have been becoming more common, but that is uncertain. More likely, the rapidly increasing scientific interest in the nature of diseases in the latter half of the eighteenth century, encouraged in Sweden by the famous physician and botanist, Linnaeus, had seized on this arresting and challenging disease for further description and discussion.

One of the best accounts was written by a Finnish medical student, A. R. Martin. He divided the progression of the disease into the customary three stages. First, general malaise and loss of weight, nodules under the skin of forehead, eyebrows, cheeks, neck, and limbs; raised, uneven patches on the skin, which ulcerated and exuded fluid, leaving a leaden-blue lump with rough, fissured skin. Second, lumps all over the feet with swelling of feet and legs, even nodules on the white of the eye itself. Finally, severe involvement of nose, nodulation and ulceration around the lips "so that it appears that the flesh will fall out", and a hoarse and a hissing voice. Surprisingly, he did not refer to disease of the nerves, but he did emphasise the chronicity of the disease, saying that twelve to fourteen years may elapse before the advanced stage is reached.

Isaac Uddman, son of a merchant in the Finnish town Kristinestad, defended the first M.D. thesis on leprosy before Linnaeus at the university of Uppsala. He became the first to predict that the shape the disease takes depends not only on its duration, but on the constitution of the individual—a fact which has recently become central to understanding of the variability of the disease. He also observed that it "hardly ever remits spontaneously", correctly implying that spontaneous cures do rarely happen, a fundamental consideration when assessing the efficacy of treatment. The scientific interest of his concise and brilliantly argued work is not relevant here, but it should be mentioned that seventy-five years before Henle propounded a detailed theory of infection by microbes, Uddman wrote

> "... we are hardly able to draw any other conclusion other than that each of these feverish illnesses such as plague, smallpox, measles, syphilis ... have their own small animals of almost infinitesimal smallness". (4)

He went on to suggest that the causative organism of leprosy would be found in the skin nodules "if ever there were access to the corpse of a leper". "In this way", he continued, "it will become possible to devise a new method more sure than hitherto, to cure the disease." The causative bacillus was first identified in the contents of a leprous nodule more than a century later.

A case report by J. L. Odhelius of Stockholm in 1774 is also important. Its interest does not reside so much in the description of a girl with a gruff, harsh voice, and with dark coloured nodules on face and limbs, as in the fact that Odhelius worked at the Seraphimer hospital, the hospital to which Ålander islanders used to go for medical diagnosis. There is no reason to suppose that the Seraphimer hospital had changed its criteria for the diagnosis in the intervening years.

The long tradition of leprosy in Iceland crystallised into objective description at this time in a monograph by Jón Petersen who was still a medical student at Copenhagen university. His clear description of leprosy was confirmed by Dr. Holland who, early in the next century, wrote from his own experience that "the leprosy of the Icelanders exhibits all the essential characteristics of genuine elephantiasis, or *lepra Arabum*, and is a disease of a most formidable and distressing kind" (5). The pearl in Petersen's long work is a letter he had recently received from a priest in Iceland, who had recognised in himself the disease he was expected to diagnose in others. This priest wrote to his medical student friend abroad in 1767 to see if he had heard of any new treatment for his incurable disease.

> "My disease, which Landphysicus Biarne Poulsen calls *Dispositionem Scorbutico Leprosam*, is progressing relentlessly. Three years ago I developed scabies on both hands and feet, which continued until last winter when it disappeared. In its place small lumps have appeared on my feet, upper legs, arms, and face. My face is becoming swollen, but it has not yet become bluish or dark. ... In ... my upper leg I have lost all sensation, so that one could easily put a hot or cold iron upon it without feeling it. The loss of sensation is equally profound on the soles of my feet. I cannot yet complain of difficulty in breathing, although my voice has become weaker. But what troubles me most at present is severe and almost insufferable pain in my feet so that I can scarcely bear to stay in bed." (6)

The mixture of skin, voice, and nervous manifestations of leprosy was no surprise to the Icelandic priest, nor for that matter to the parish priests of Norway, because in isolated communities all serious illness tends to land on the priest's doorstep. Pastor Strøm described ten cases of leprosy amongst his parishioners in Bolden, West Norway, between 1764 and 1774. His diagnosis was confirmed medically in three who ended their days at the Reknæs leper hospital, Molde. One of his parishioners, a 20-year-old man by the name of Torvig, attributed the onset of his disease to sleeping out in the fields on a cold night without shoes when drunk after a wedding; three or four years later, he was taken to the leper hospital. Another, a 19-year-old boy called Selbervig, had had symptoms including itching and loss of sensation for nearly eight years before he was taken to hospital. Strøm mentions all the characteristic signs in face, nose, voice, and limbs, and insists that this disease cannot easily be confused with any other. Weddings in his parish were clearly gay events, for he mentions another young man whom he suspected to have leprosy, whose disease seemed to have dated from dancing at a wedding "until sweat dropped off him". In the parish of Bolden the young men suffered from the exhaustion of attending weddings and the maidens from the frustration of not being personally involved. Strøm had come across one case, and heard of another in a neighbouring parish, of young women who, "because of grief over their fiancé's unfaithfulness, first fell into a frenzy, and soon after became leprous".

The fullest, most discerning, and accurate pre-scientific description of leprosy was also written by a priest, Pastor Welhaven of Bergen. In 1816, he published in the journal of the Swedish Medical Association an account which would have done credit to any doctor. His critical insight may well have been the inspiration to *Om Spedalskhed*, the first scientific monograph on the clinical and pathological features of leprosy, which was published in Bergen by D. C. Danielssen and C. W. Boeck in 1847. Their work not only founded the scientific study of leprosy, but marked the beginning of a tradition of leprosy research in Bergen, which culminated in the discovery of the causative bacillus by Hansen in 1873 (7).

Wellhaven's descriptions are the climax of centuries of untutored observation of this strange disease:

> "Leprosy manifests itself in some people as a variable number of larger and smaller violet-red lumps. After one or more years they develop into round corroding sores which do not heal. ... In some the disease appears only as bluish or dark-red spots on the face and body. The chest is affected by a hoarseness which makes the breath short and speech incomprehensible ... they as it were, suffocate with viscous phlegm ... which obstructs the windpipe, deprives them of breath and causes a dry cough, which in its outburst severely exhausts the patient.... The country people call this suffocating hoarseness 'kiove'....
>
> "Some do not have any skin nodules but they nevertheless have indubitable characteristics of leprosy ... Their eyebrows soon fall out, and a strange lameness is experienced in their limbs and joints, which resembles that after a stroke, and they experience severe pain in their legs. ...
>
> "Many with leprosy become completely blind. ...
>
> "It is also not uncommon for the small digits of fingers and toes of many with this gnawing disease to fall off, as the disease gnaws and consumes these unfortunate people to marrow and bone. ...
>
> "Some show the disease plainly in their feet which are deformed, crooked and disabled, and much resemble elephants' legs, being rounded off at the toes so that those can hardly be seen. ..."

Only thirty years in time, and nothing in spirit, separates Welhaven's account and discussion of the disease from its scientific dawn in *Om Spedalskhed*. His is the last and firmest link in a long chain of description linking medieval to modern times.

2. *Pictorial evidence*

No proof of leprosy can be expected from pictures before the nineteenth century. Throughout the Middle Ages pictorial illustration of scientific works was strictly diagrammatic. The herbals of Brunfels (1530) and Fuchs (1542) were the first biological books to have lifelike illustrations, and at about the same time anatomical illustration also adopted a realism founded on accurate observation, notably in *De Fabrica Humani Corporis* (1543) by Vesalius. As Hall has so cogently expressed it, "in no real sense was this the moment of the birth of some novel, self-conscious method of observation and experiment in science, but it was the moment when the accepted narrative of fact and theory was first modified effectively and permanently by recourse to nature" (8). Nearly another three centuries elapsed before the understanding of disease was challenged and enhanced by naturalistic illustration.

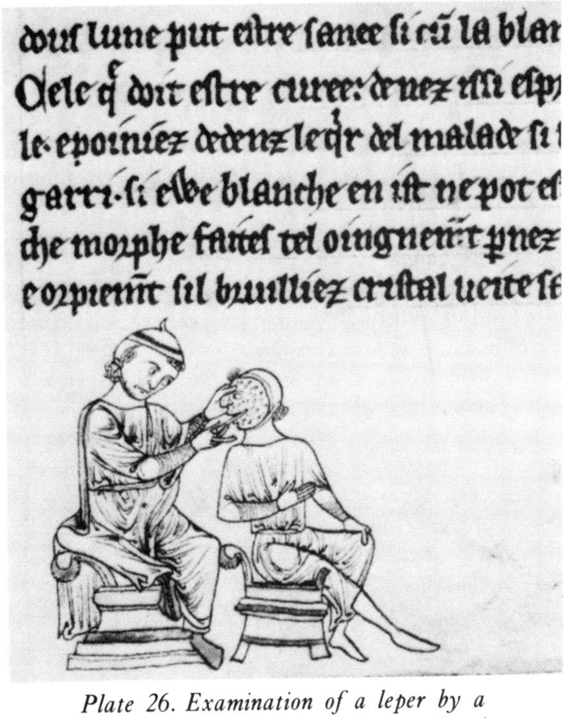

Plate 26. Examination of a leper by a physician: marginal sketch in a medieval manuscript belonging to Trinity College, Cambridge.

Artists themselves were busy with other more distinguished, handsome, and remunerative subjects than the victims of leprosy. What possible incentive had they to draw a penniless and disfigured leper, except perhaps as background to a scene of noble charity? Deformed and horrible beggars do appear in this rôle, but such licence was used in portraying their appearance that even if leprosy inspired their nightmarish appearance no certain medical diagnosis can be made. Medieval illustration can only offer a symbolic portrayal of spotted, deformed beggars, their rattles, bells, crutches, and begging bowls (Plates 15, 16, 26, 27)—

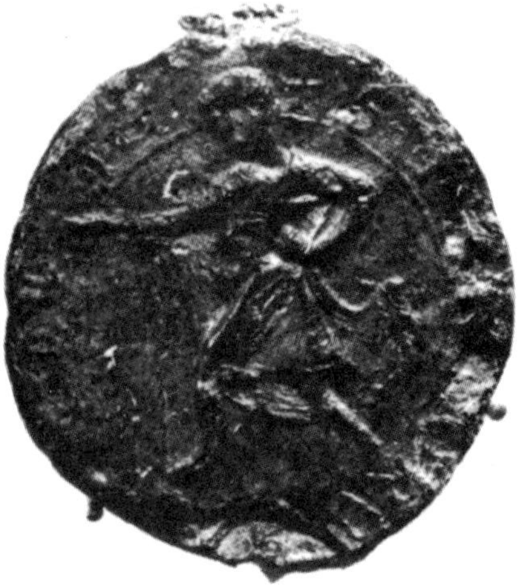

Plate 27. Impression of the late twelfth-century seal of the leper hospital of the Holy Innocents, Lincoln. The beggar's outstretched right arm is supported by an elbow crutch and his left hand is holding a shoulder crutch.

the "unclene spotyd" lepers covered with "reddie Whelkes and Pymples". These permit no diagnosis, but it is hard to resist the conviction that the monk who painted the lifelike spotted beggar with his bell, shown in Plate 16, had painted a leper from life. His wooden leg and arm are difficult to explain, unless he had been injured in war before becoming a leper; mutilation is common in advanced leprosy but limbs are not lost.

The first person to be drawn with the purpose of proving the nature of his disease was a Shetlander, John Berns, a 28-year-old man who was admitted to the Royal Infirmary at Edinburgh in 1798 with a disease which at first defied diagnosis. His face was studded with small subcutaneous nodules, the overlying skin had a blotchy red appearance, the eyebrows and eyelashes had fallen out, and his nose was ulcerated within; his voice was weak and hoarse. The rest of his body was

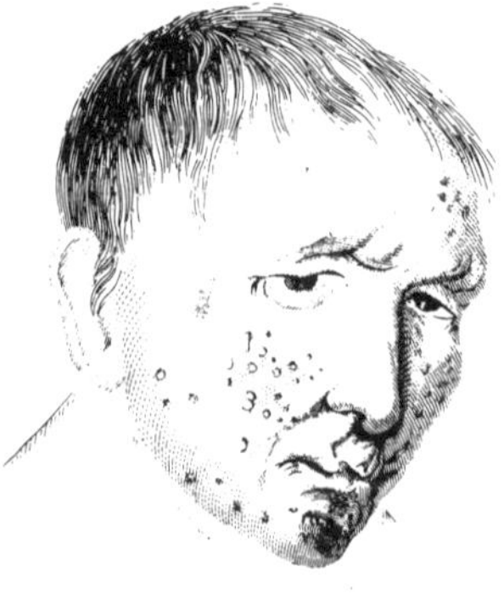

Plate 28. John Berns of Shetland, possibly the last case of endemic leprosy in the British Isles, drawn by Syme in the Royal Infirmary, Edinburgh, in 1798.

covered with small lumps under the skin. Some of his ancestors were reported to have suffered from the same disease. Dr. Thomson, who was in charge of the case, sent a sketch of the patient (Plate 28) to Robert Willan, now acclaimed the father of British dermatology. Willan declared without reservation that Berns had leprosy (9). No certain diagnosis can be made from the sketch alone, but the loss of the hair of the eyebrows, and their heavy nodulation, are suggestive. John Berns was probably the last recognised case of endemic leprosy in the British Isles.

There is no ambiguity in most of Pastor Welhaven's drawings of lepers in Bergen a few years later. Neither the identity of the disease nor his recognition of its many variations are in doubt. These sketches had long been forgotten and had never been published before the author rediscovered copies of some of them in a manuscript (10) in the University of Bergen library in 1957. A footnote to Welhaven's description of the hospital and its inmates had mentioned that twenty-eight sketches had been deposited with the Swedish Medical Society in 1816. In 1936, the managers of a fund set up with the small surplus from the Second International Leprosy Conference at Bergen in 1909 entered into negotiations with the Swedish Medical Society for permission to reproduce Welhaven's pictures, which were still in their possession. Permission was granted on the condition that the pictures did not leave Stockholm. A Stockholm artist copied the pictures and a local firm was entrusted with engraving them. The reproductions were received in Bergen and the account was duly paid.

When the leper hospital Pleistiftelse no. 1 was cleared out in 1971, a box was discovered containing reproductions of Welhaven's drawings. The originals have not been seen since 1936. As custodians of these unique sketches the Swedish Medical Society must bear a heavy responsibility for their loss. Searches at the Royal Library in Stockholm, the National Museum, the State Archives and the Medical History Museum, have all drawn a blank.

Welhaven's pictures are a milestone in both social and medical history to which full justice cannot be done here. There is no doubt that leprosy is portrayed. His

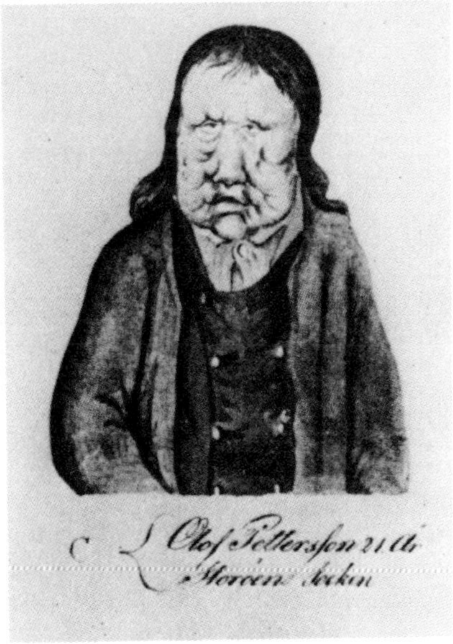

Plate 29. Olof Pettersen, aged 21, drawn by J. A. Welhaven about 1816 to show how leprosy could transform a young man into the appearance of "an evil wrinkled old man".

picture of 21-year-old Olof Petterson (Plate 29) shows how the disease could transform a young man into "an evil, wrinkled old man". The heavy nodulation of his brows, cheeks, mouth, and chin give him the classical lion-like appearance (*facies leonina*) of leprosy. The features of the face of Anna Axels Dotter (Plate

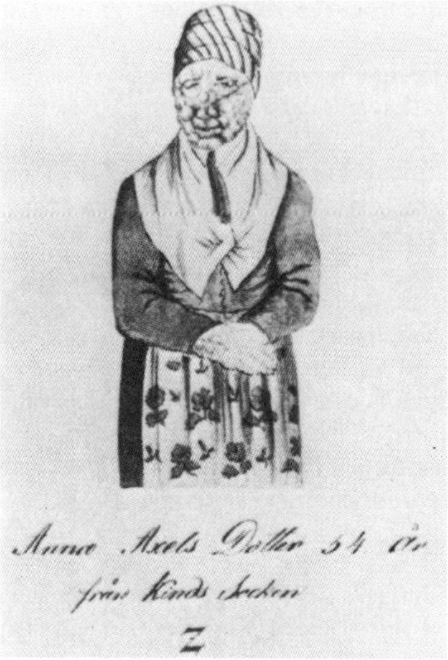

Plate 30. Anna Axels Dotter, aged 54, drawn by J. A. Welhaven to illustrate the nodular form of leprosy.

30), aged 54, are almost completely obscured by confluent bluish red nodulation of her face, and she has similar nodules on her hands closely resembling the appearance of a Finnish patient (Plate 31) diagnosed in 1945; this Finnish patient has since been cured with modern drugs. The same disease is seen at an earlier stage

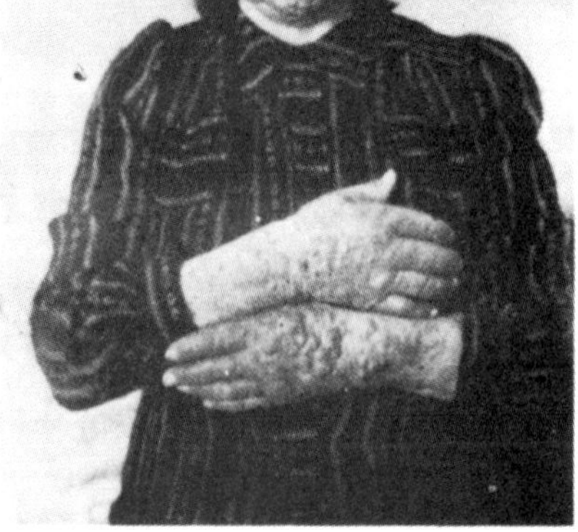

Plate 31. Nodular leprosy similar to the case of Anna Axels Dotter (and cf. Plate 41) in one of the last Finnish patients when diagnosed in 1945.

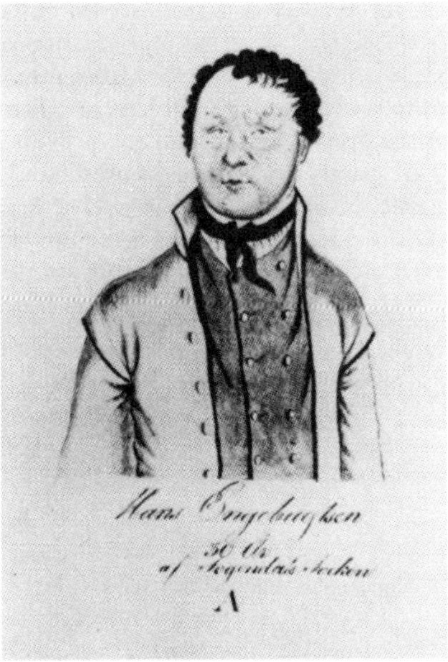

Plate 32. Hans Engebugtsen, aged 30, drawn by J. A. Welhaven to illustrate early nodular leprosy.

in the face of Hans Engebugsten (Plate 32), aged 30, who was "an extremely dashing soldier in the campaign of 1808, when he noticed a hard lump over his left eyebrow where he had been struck by a stray bullet at the battle of Jerpset. Soon after his home-coming from the war the disease broke out in small nodules on his feet which developed into sores: later similar lumps appeared on his face." He has nodules around his eyebrows and small superficial reddish brown papules on his forehead, around his nose, and on his upper lip; his eyebrows have lost their hair.

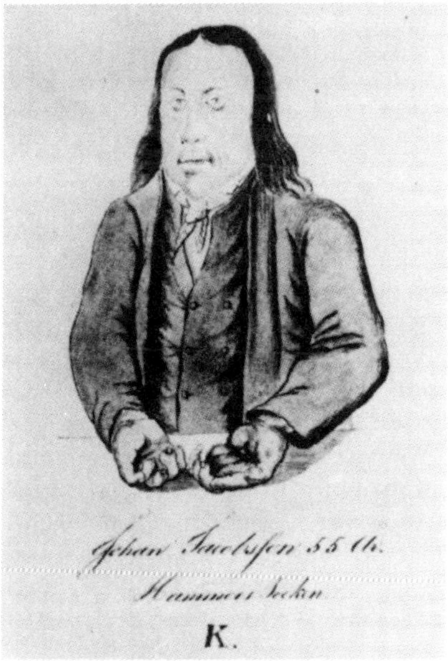

Plate 33. Johan Jacobssen, aged 55, drawn by J. A. Welhaven as an example of paralysis of face and hands caused by leprosy from which he had suffered for 27 years; his fingers are becoming shortened.

The disease had not yet sapped his strength, for Welhaven describes him as "a strong, diligent, and hard-working fellow".

Johan Jacobssen (Plate 33) is important because his picture proves that leprosy was known sometimes to destroy nerves without causing the characteristic skin disease. He also exemplifies the chronicity of the disease better than any previous report. Both sides of his expressionless face are paralysed, and his clawed hands with stubby, shortened fingers are characteristic. Jacobbsen experienced the first symptoms of his disease "like a needle prick in his left thumb" when he was 28 years old, twenty-seven years before Welhaven etched his sad appearance on the canvas of history. Anna Nils Dotter (Plate 34), aged 64, shows the same form

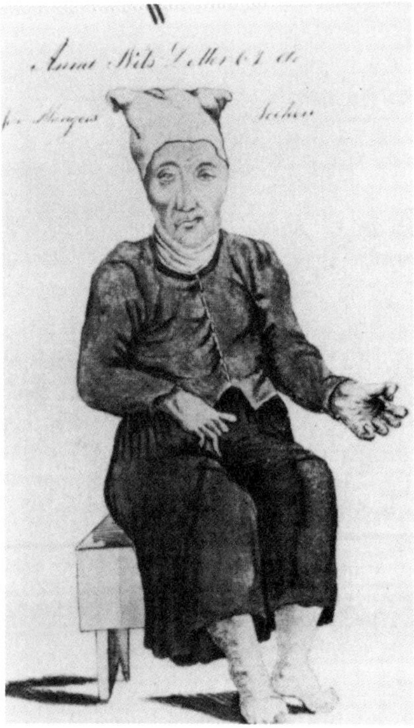

Plate 34. Anna Nils Dotter, aged 64, showing leprosy in the same form as in Johan Jacobssen (Plate 46) but also with swelling of her legs and mutilation of her toes.

of the disease: both sides of her face are paralysed, both hands are clawed, and her toes are both shortened and mutilated; she is also blind.

Iceland, a country settled by Norwegians in the ninth century, preserved a continuous tradition of leprosy throughout many centuries of relative isolation. Petersen and his tragic friend the priest leave no doubt from their descriptions that the same disease simmered on in Iceland as in Scandinavia itself. In 1835-36, a French scientific expedition visited Iceland and Greenland aboard the corvette *La Recherche*. They published several volumes of geological, topographical, and biological observations together with two volumes of plates (11), which included eight lepers: seven are the work of the artist L. Bevalet and the eighth is by the expedition's doctor, E. Robert. Altogether fourteen cases of leprosy were described and discussed in the volume on zoology and medicine. Long forgotten, these portraits show in Iceland the same disease that Welhaven had documented twenty years before in Norway.

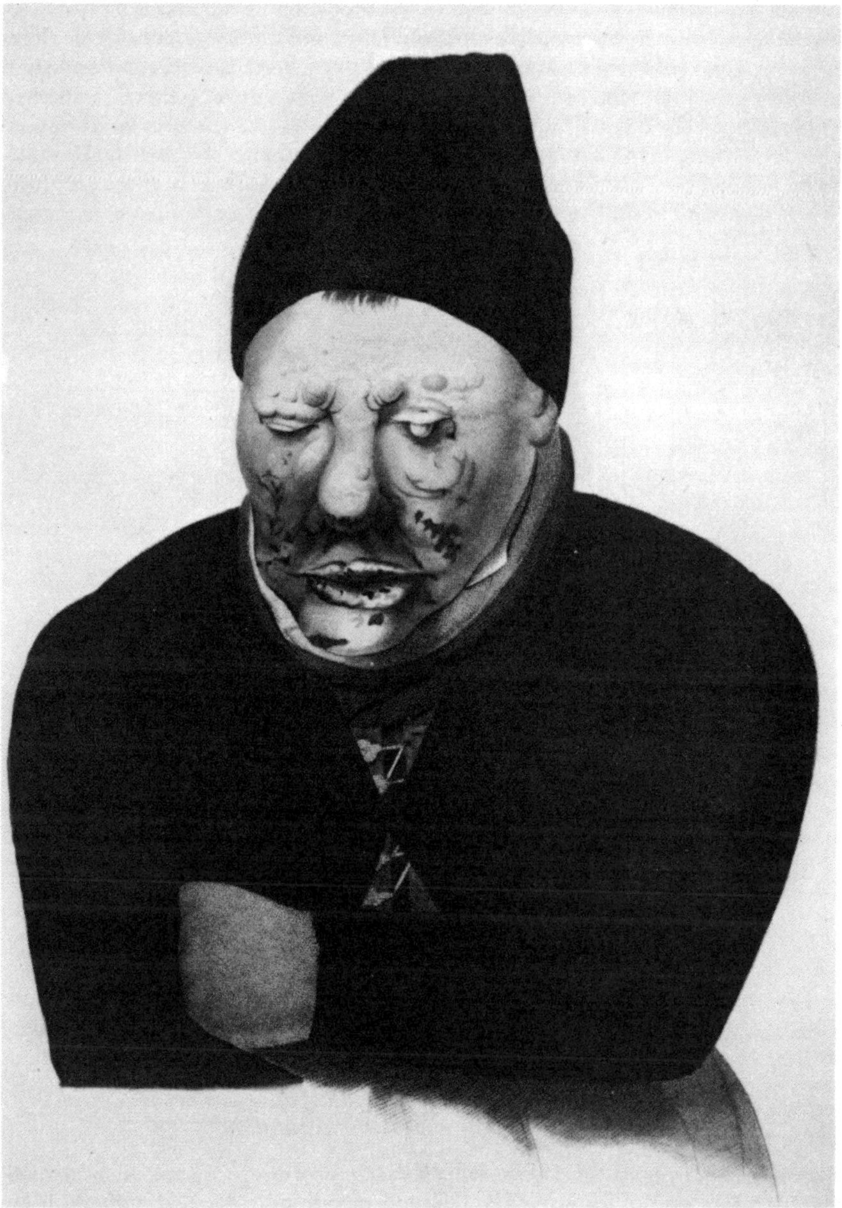

Plate 35. Rósa Olafsdottir, aged 68, of Mödrufell, Iceland, drawn by Bevalet in 1836. She was described as the "most repulsive" case of leprosy that the expedition encountered. Although suffering thus for more than twenty years she was singing while this picture was drawn.

Rósa Olafsdóttir of Mödrufell (Plate 35), aged 68, described as the "most repulsive" case the expedition encountered, is depicted in semi-diagrammatic form. Did the horror of the sight prove too much for the artist, so that he fled before completing his picture? Leprous nodules are recognisable on both eyebrows with loss of their hair, she has a nodule on her left eye, and nodules and fissured ulcers on nose, lips, cheeks, and chin; she is blind. Robert records with admiration and astonishment that "she did not seem overcome with sorrow", although she had suffered from the disease for more than twenty years, and was now so disfigured that the features of her face were hardly recognisable and her feet were badly mutilated. Lesser, but nevertheless characteristic, nodular swellings over the eyebrows are evident in Sniólfúr Thorleifson (Plate 36), aged 40, whose leprous wife, Arndis

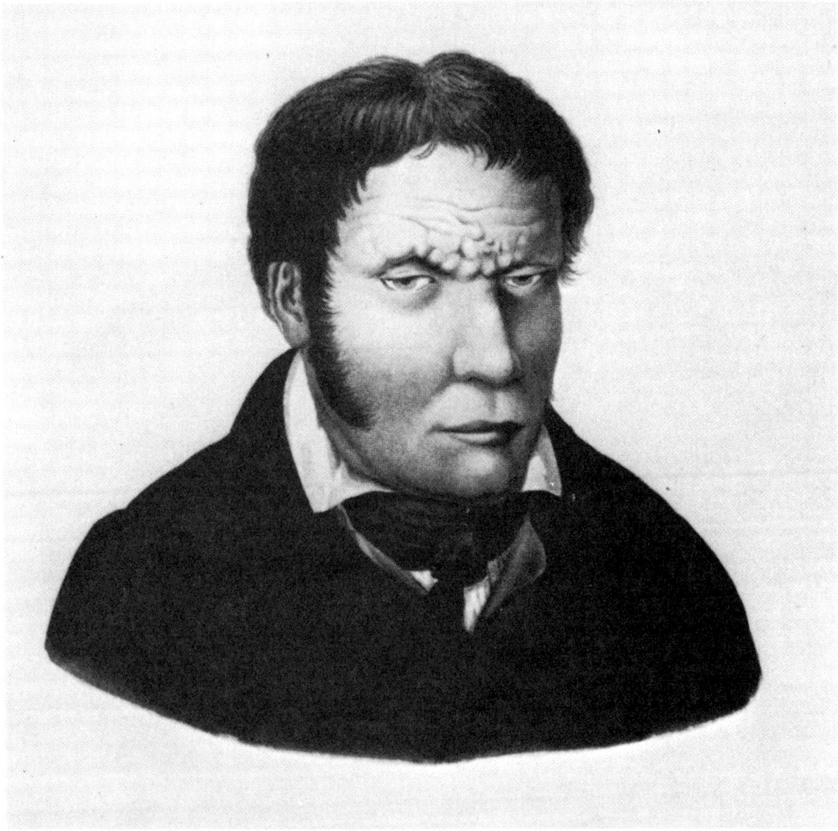

Plate 36. Sniólfúr Thorleifson, aged 40, of Nes, Iceland, drawn by Bevalet in 1836 to show leprous nodules on his forehead.

Einarsdóttir, was also sketched when Robert and Bevalet visited them at their home at Nes on July 22nd, 1836. Thorleifson's grandfather had suffered from the same disease, but his parents had been healthy. Icelandic doctors, no less than Welhaven, recognised blindness and destruction of nerves as features of leprosy: Finnur Jónsson (Plate 37), aged 34, of Thingvellir, has been left with his face paralysed and his eyes blind.

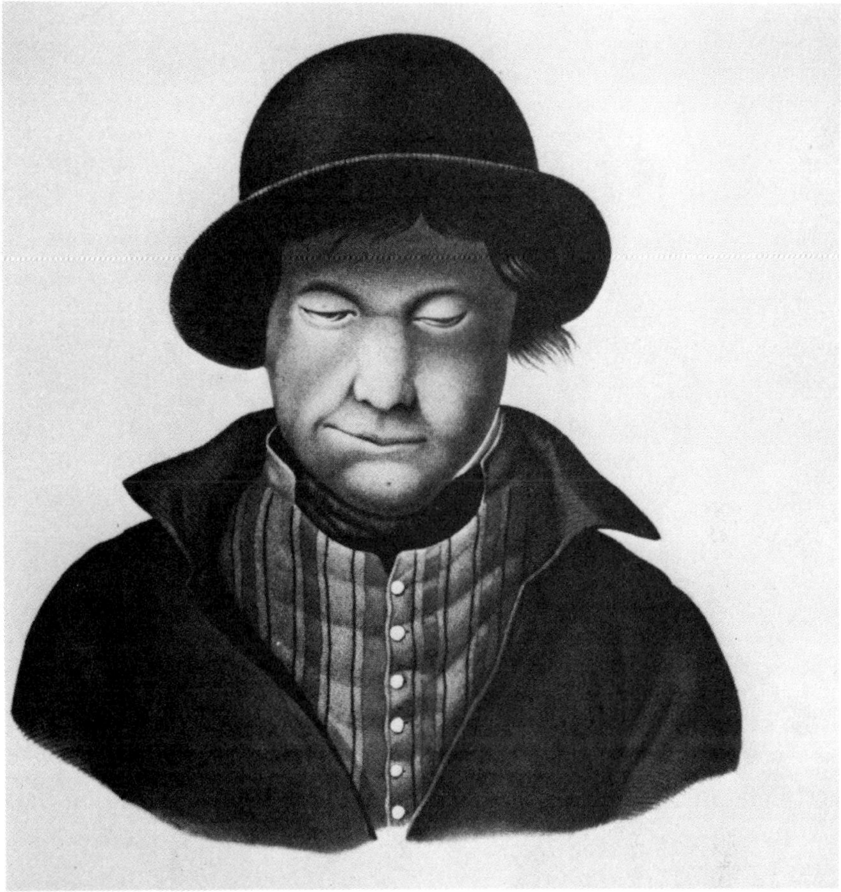

Plate 37. Finnur Jönsson, aged 34, of Thingvellir, Iceland, drawn by Bevalet in 1836 to show paralysis of the face and blindness as a result of leprosy.

It is generally agreed that the plates in Danielssen and Boeck's *Atlas* of 1847 portray leprosy. The resemblance between the disease they illustrate and that drawn by Welhaven and by Bevalet is unmistakable. A 13-year-old boy, leprous since the age of 6 (Plate 38), is shown with extensive and characteristic brownish-red nodulation of his face and ears, contrasting with his bright blue coat and neckerchief. A sad young woman in a blue bonnet and pink shawl (Plate 39) has nodules on her eyebrows and on the right eye itself, and the right side of her face is paralysed. The fearsome appearance of the disease is brought home by the distorted, partly paralysed face of one young man (Plate 40) and by the grossly nodulated, crusted face and blind left eye of a 28-year-old woman (Plate 41), as satyr-like as any medieval leper. These portraits remove any doubt that the difficulty with which disfigured Cresseid was recognised was an unreal flight of poetical fancy.

Gaps there were in the knowledge of leprosy, and many enigmas still remain after another 130 years of research. But these pictures match the first medieval descriptions of leprosy, and leave no doubt that the most obvious cases of the

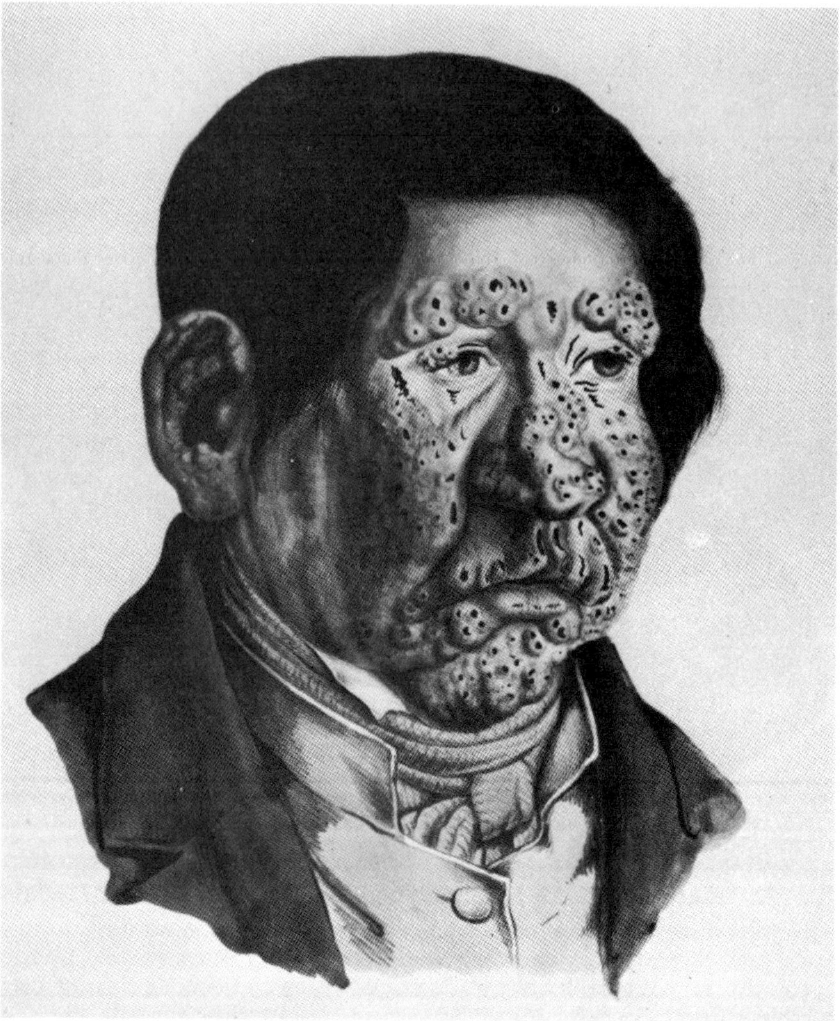

Plate 38. A 13-year-old boy with nodular leprosy for seven years, from Danielssen and Boeck (1847).

disease were correctly recognised. Ordinary people were familiar with the characteristic features of the disease. The traditions passed on from century to century by priests and people were not improved on by doctors for more than 500 years.

3. *Graveyard proof*

Words are open to many interpretations; pictures show only one brief moment in time, and their value as evidence is limited by the artist's skill, understanding, and licence. Is there no more objective evidence that the historical traditions of leprosy are scientifically sound? Leprosy mutilates if the sufferer lives long enough, and bones degenerate along with the flesh. Changes in the bones of hands

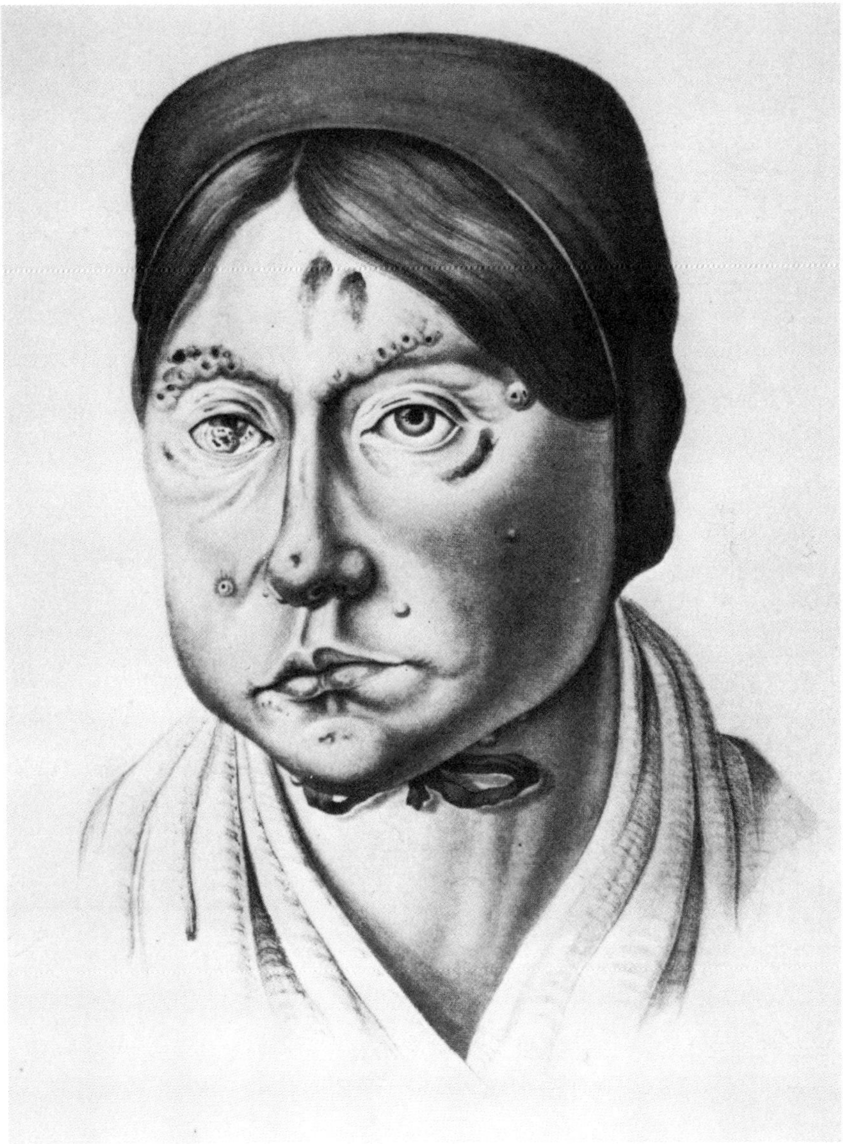

Plate 39. Nodular leprosy and right facial paralysis in a 26-year-old woman, from Danielssen and Boeck (1847).

and feet have been recognised on X-ray photographs for years. Could these mutilations not be found in the bones of medieval lepers?

Chance happenings lack significance to those without memory or imagination. But to those with the gift of seeing much in little, the most inconsequential events may become the springboard to new discoveries. In 1944, when excavating the site of the large Augustinian monastery at Æbelholt, about 30 miles north of

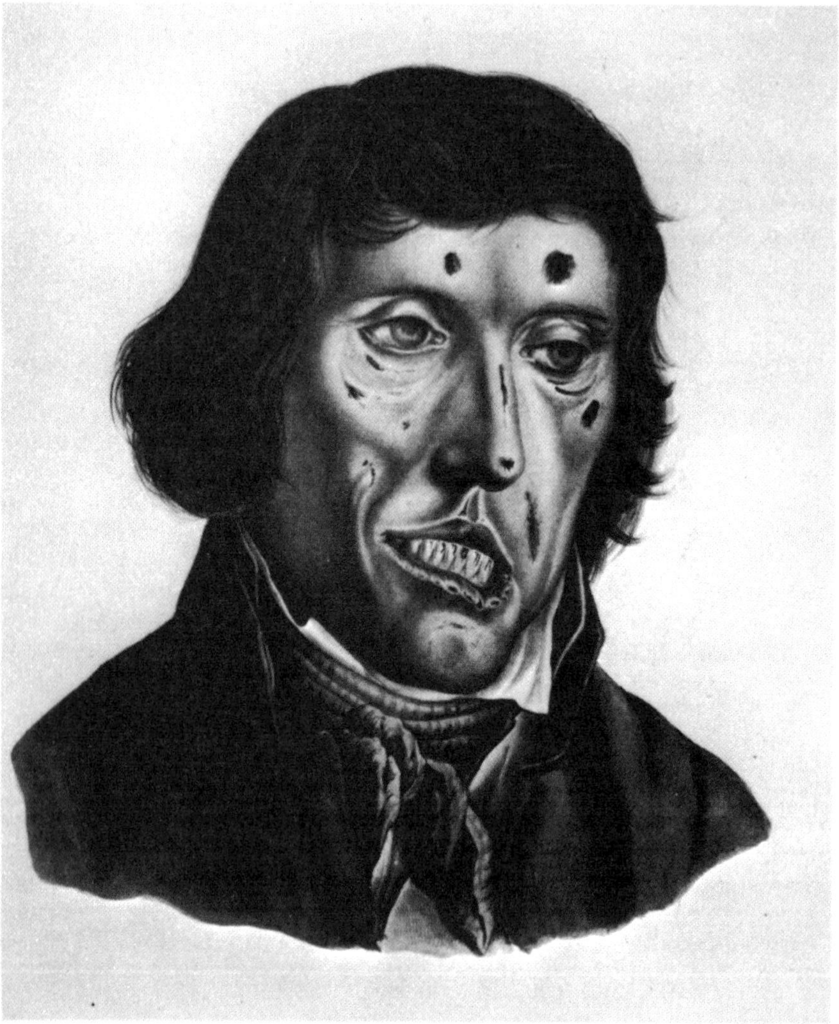

Plate 40. A 38-year-old man whose face has become paralysed as a result of leprosy, from Danielssen and Boeck (1847).

Copenhagen, V. Møller-Christensen, a general practitioner who later became professor of the history of medicine at Copenhagen, discovered a skeleton with deformities he could not identify. Professors from Copenhagen and Oslo were also puzzled. In retrospect, the changes were probably those of chronic ergotism ("St. Anthony's Fire"), but leprosy was one of the possibilities considered at the time. The difficulty was that no one knew what the bones of a leper might look like after several hundred years in Danish soil.

Møller-Christensen then recalled a spring day in 1929 when, as a young assistant at the hospital at Næstved, a town about 50 miles south west of Copenhagen, he

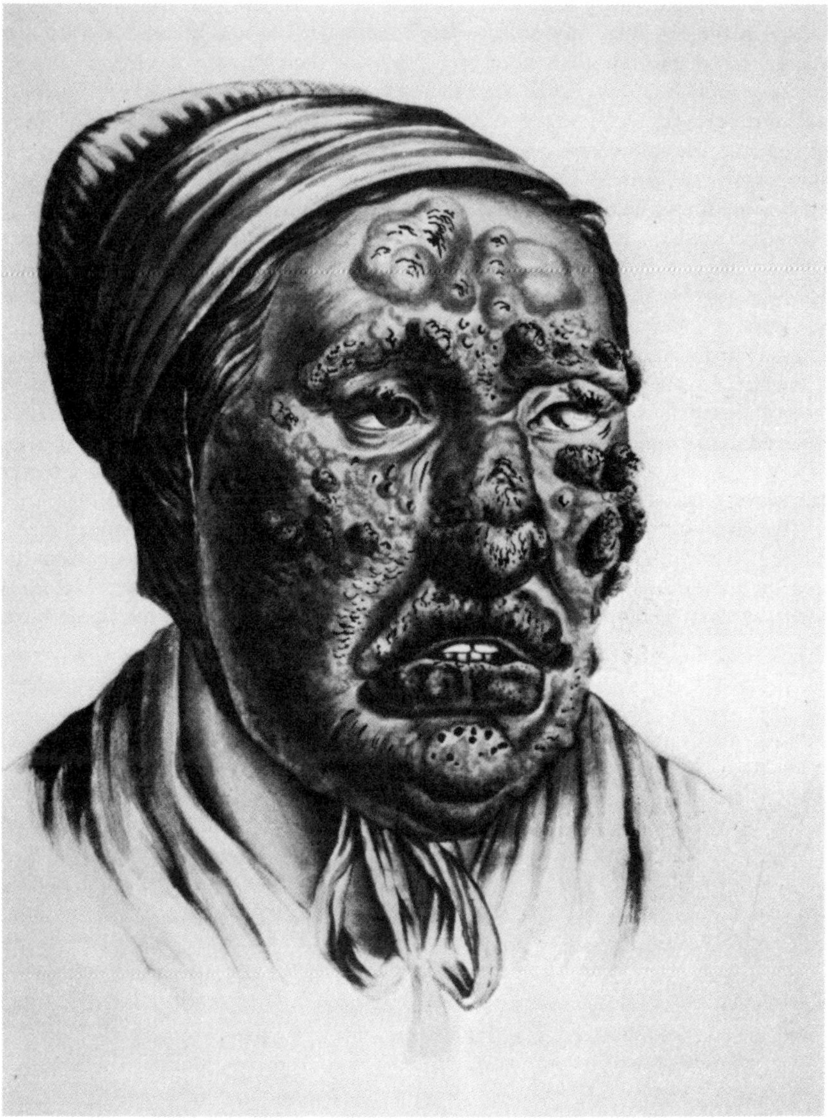

Plate 41. Extensive nodular leprosy in a 28-year-old woman, from Danielssen and Boeck (1847).

had driven out with his chief to see a patient. They had paused for a moment by the small village of Åderup on the outskirts of the town. Pointing to meadows by the river, his colleague showed him the traditional site of the medieval St. George's leper hospital of Næstved. Now, twenty years later, Møller-Christensen turned over in his mind the slender possibility that the leper hospital of Næstved might hold the key to his undiagnosed skeleton.

One Sunday in August, 1948, Møller-Christensen set out for Næstved. His hopes and expectations were quickly dashed, for on the peaceful meadows of twenty years ago there now stood a large factory. That was the end of that—or was it? Local traditions are often right, but only half-right: if tradition were in this case a few hundred yards out, the lepers might yet lie undisturbed. Farmers talk, and no subject is better for rumour, gossip, and speculation than the discovery of human bones. Møller-Christensen made a round of the nearby farms: half a dozen surprised farmers shook their heads before he heard that human skulls had been turned up when a new drain was dug some years before on a farm about 500 yards south of the traditional site of the hospital. The farm-house had been built in the last century on land belonging to the Næstved almshouses. Land belonging to leper hospitals had in the sixteenth century been transferred to local hospitals or other charities; this seemed a promising lead.

The farmer was aware of an old tradition that his farm had been built on a graveyard for the poor. Indeed it was a graveyard, but not merely for the poor. A preliminary dig that year and more extensive excavations in 1950 and 1951 uncovered many skeletons, most of which were mutilated in a fashion never seen before in medieval skeletons (12). The walls of a late gothic church with a tower at the west end were also found, the remains of the hospital's church.

These and subsequent excavations in, around, and under the four-winged farmhouse (Plates 42, 43) have yielded 202 skeletons or skulls in sufficiently good condition for a diagnosis of leprosy to be confirmed or denied (13). Besides skeletons showing classical deformities of hands and feet, three quarters of the skulls show

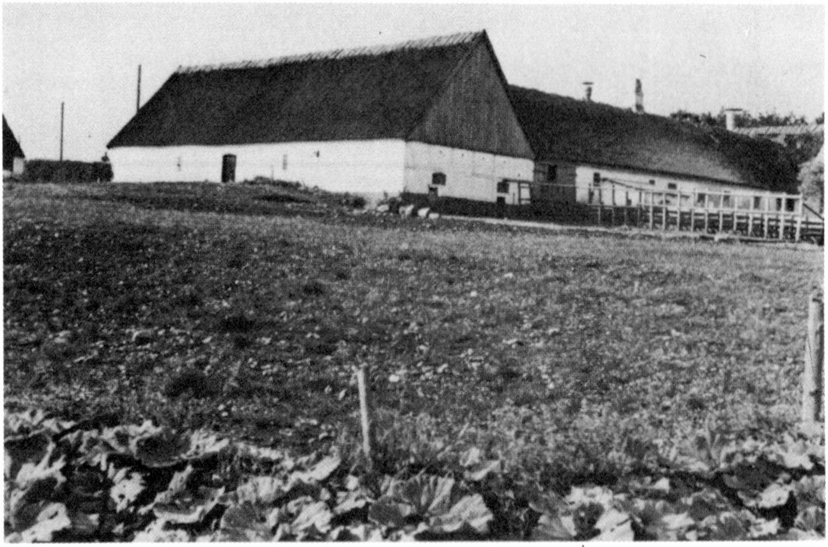

Plate 42. The farm built on the site of the medieval leper graveyard at Næstved, Denmark.

evidence of severe infection within the nose, together with either or both atrophy of the anterior nasal spine (14) and atrophy of the central part of the alveolar margin of the maxillary bone, resulting in loosening or loss of the upper incisor teeth. In Plate 44 both the anterior nasal spine and the alveolar margin of the maxilla have been eroded, and the teeth have fallen out. In contrast, Plate 45 shows gross

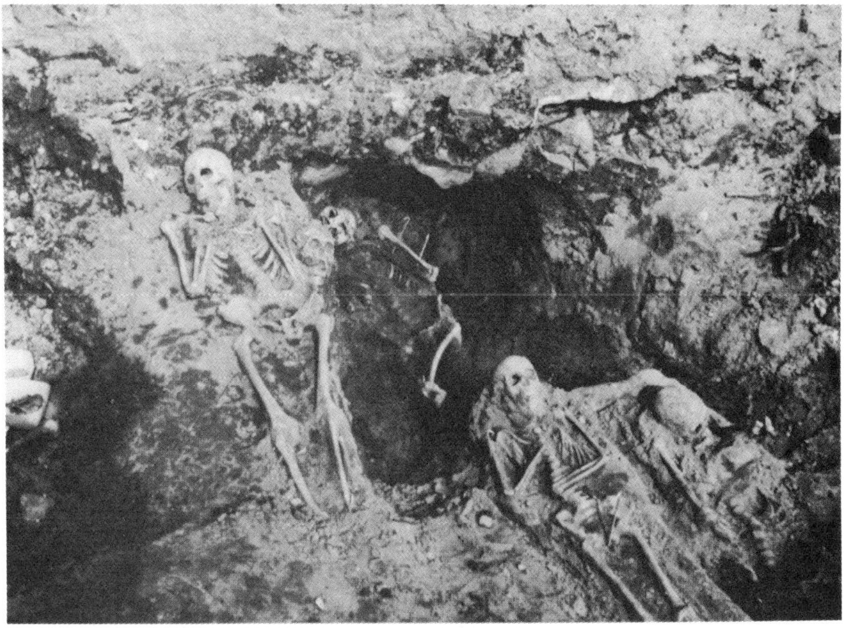

Plate 43. Medieval lepers of Næstved during the excavation of 1957.

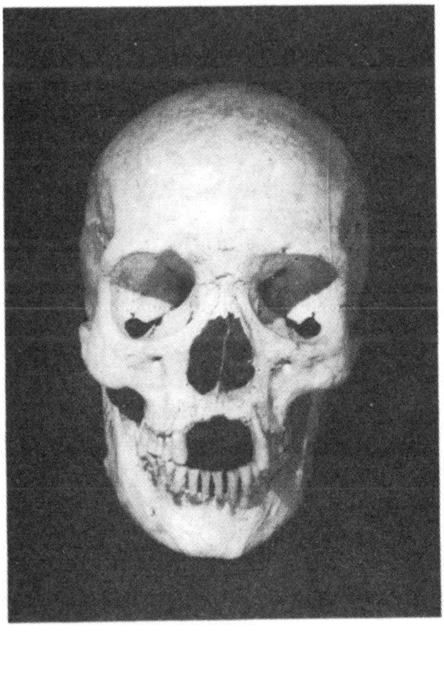

Plate 44. The only skull from Øm monastery, Denmark, which showed leprous changes. The central part of the alveolar margin of the maxillary bone has atrophied and the anterior nasal spine has disappeared.

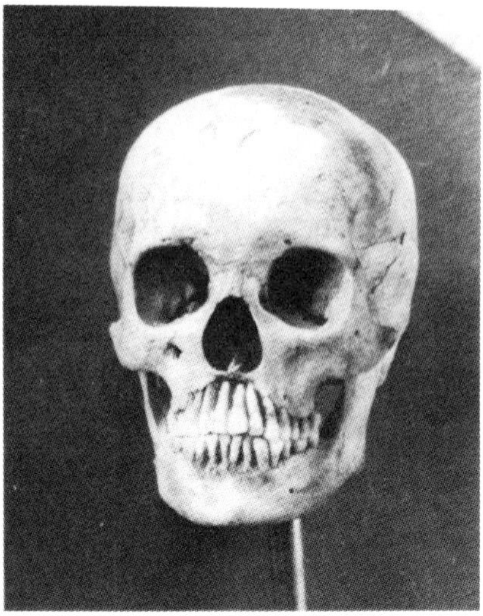

Plate 45. Leprous changes in a skull from Næstved leper graveyard. The teeth have not been lost but the maxillary atrophy is similar to that in Plate 44. The anterior nasal spine is preserved.

erosion of the alveolar margin without loss of teeth; the anterior nasal spine is still preserved.

These changes in the skull, which Møller-Christensen named *facies leprosa*, had not been suspected in living lepers, although destruction of tissues within and around the nose has long been recognised as a feature of the disease. The medieval lepers of Næstved have taught twentieth century medicine a lesson: identical skull pathology has since been detected radiologically in 5 out of 8 lepers (62%) in Norway (15), 57 out of 96 (59%) in Belgian Congo (16), and in 40 out of 56 (71%) in India (17). An independent examination of the Næstved skeletons by J. G. Andersen in 1969 reached a definite diagnosis of leprosy in 155 out of 202 individuals (77%) buried in and around the chapel of St. George's hospital at Næstved (17). No other disease is known today which could account for the skull changes. Other diseases may rarely cause similar deformities of hands and feet, but the combination with the skull pathology leaves no reasonable doubt that the Næstved disease was leprosy. Taking into account the fact that leprosy does not invariably damage bones, it seems certain that the majority of those buried at Næstved were lepers.

Is there any alternative explanation? Might the soil at Næstved, for example, have caused a peculiar weathering of these skeletons? If so, it would be difficult to explain why the anterior nasal spine of some skulls is perfectly preserved and the alveolar margin of the maxilla is badly eroded, while in others the reverse is true; and in the remainder (amounting to about one quarter of the total) the skull is well preserved in both respects. Nevertheless, erosion in the grave might conceivably explain why *facies leprosa* was common at Næstved and absent from 760 medieval skulls at Æbelholt monastery (18). But it would not explain the presence of just one skull with identical and severe changes amongst 633 medieval burials at Øm monastery (Plate 44) the skeleton of which individual was the only one there to show mutilations of hands and feet (19). This one case of leprosy in the graveyard of Øm monastery is an enigma. It is unlikely that her disease was not recognised, because she would surely have been obviously and characteristically disfigured. She was, however, buried in the deepest (and therefore oldest) layer of the cemetery, which was in use from 1172. The most probably explanation is that she was buried before the decree of 1179 that lepers should be interred in separate graveyards. Alternatively, she may have obtained the special permission allowed under that decree for a leper to be buried in a general graveyard.

If the bone disease at Næstved cannot be explained by erosion in the soil, could it not be attributed instead to a disease unknown or rare today but common then? A disease as mysterious, perhaps, as the Sweating Sickness, which first broke out in England in 1485, recurred in four more impressive and well-documented epidemics in 1508, 1517, 1528 and 1551, and then vanished without trace (20). It really would be incredible if any hypothetical disfiguring disease were to have been confined by chance to Næstved, affected at least 77% of those buried in one particular graveyard over a period of four hundred years, yet appeared only once in nearly fourteen hundred burials in two Danish monastery graveyards during the same period, one of which is less than 100 miles away.

Furthermore, there is a distinct and impressive difference in the other diseases found in these medieval graveyards. Monasteries were the only general hospitals in the Middle Ages, and sixty people (mostly men) buried at Øm (21) and Æbelholt (22) had injuries caused by axe, sword, spear, and other weapons; at Næstved, traumatic injuries were noticeable by their absence. Several other diseases, including septic infections of bones, tuberculosis, and cancer are found at the monasteries, but not at Næstved. Syphilis, a disease, which, on controversial evidence, some historians have said was mistaken for leprosy (23), causes characteristic destruction of bone: it has been found in a handful of skeletons from both of the

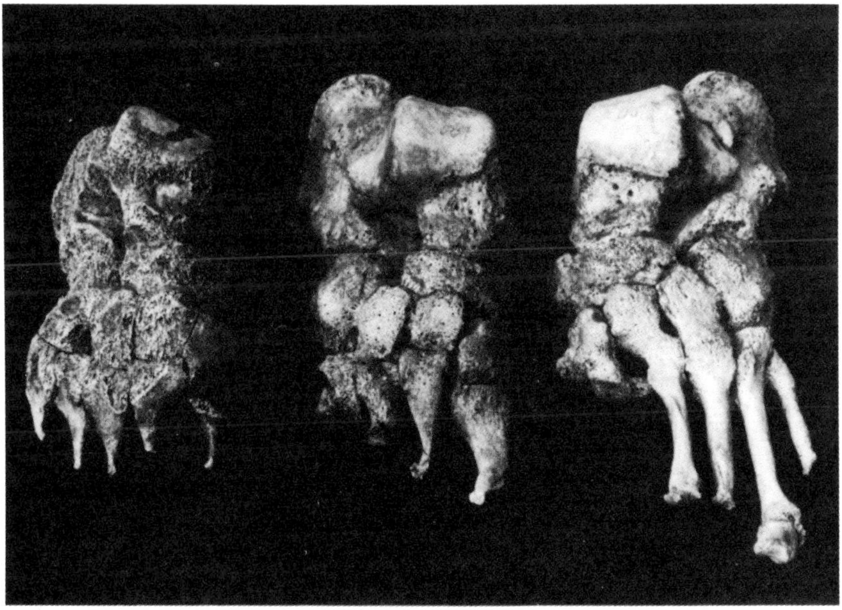

Plate 46. Bones of feet mutilated by leprosy found in the medieval leper graveyards at Næstved and Svendborg.

large monasteries, all of them in the most recent burial layers dating from about 1500–60, but it has not been found at Næstved.

To prove conclusively that the people buried at Næstved belonged to the leper hospital it was necessary to excavate the graveyard of another leper hospital. A small excavation was carried out in 1961 by Olav Olsen of the National Museum of Denmark at the only surviving leper hospital chapel in Denmark, St. George's church in Svendborg. Only nine skeletons were sufficiently well-preserved for a firm diagnosis to be made: they *all* showed characteristic *facies leprosa*, mutilation of the limbs (Plate 46), or both (24).

Medieval tradition records that lepers lived and were buried apart. It also tells how they lived and how they died. The skeletons of those who died in two medieval leper hospitals prove that most were indeed lepers; the absence of leprosy from two contemporary monastery graveyards confirms that advanced leprosy was correctly recognised. The medieval leper was as real as his disease.

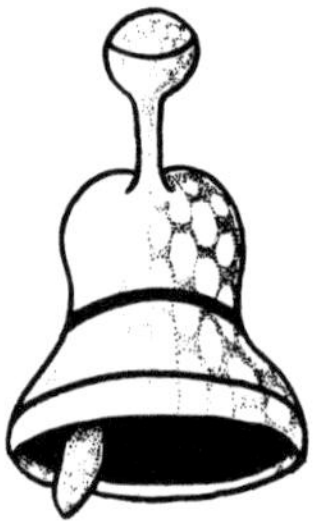

DOCUMENTS

1. Office at the seclusion of a leper.[1]

The manner of casting out or separating those who are sick with leprosy from the whole.

First of all the sick man or the leper clad in a cloak and in his usual dress, being in his house, ought to have notice of the coming of the priest who is on his way to the house to lead him to the church, and must in that guise wait for him. For the priest vested in surplice and stole, with the cross going before, makes his way to the sick man's house and addresses him with comforting words, pointing out and proving that if he blesses and praises God, and bears his sickness patiently, he may have a sure and certain hope that though he is sick in body he may be whole in soul, and may obtain the gift of everlasting salvation. And then with other words suitable to the occasion let the priest lead the leper to the church, when he has sprinkled him with holy water, the cross going before, the priest following, and last of all the sick man. Within the church let a black cloth, if it can be had, be set upon two trestles at some distance apart before the altar, and let the sick man take his place on bended knees beneath it between the trestles, after the manner of a dead man, although by the grace of God he yet lives in body and spirit, and in this posture let him devoutly hear mass. When this is finished and he has been sprinkled with holy water, he must be led with the cross through the presbytery to a place where a pause must be made. When the spot is reached the priest shall counsel him out of holy scripture, saying: "Remember thine end and thou shalt never do amiss." Whence Augustine says: "He readily esteems all things lightly, who ever bears in mind that he will die." The priest then with the spade casts earth on each of his feet, saying: "Be thou dead to the world, but alive again unto God."

And he comforts him and strengthens him to endure with the words of Isaiah spoken concerning our Lord Jesus Christ:—"Truly He hath borne our griefs and carried our sorrows, yet did we esteem Him as a leper smitten of God and afflicted." Let him say also: "If in weakness of body by means of suffering thou art made like unto Christ, thou mayest surely hope that thou wilt rejoice in spirit with God. May the Most High grant this to thee, numbering thee among his faithful ones in the book of life. Amen."

It is to be noted that the priest must lead him to the church and from the church to his house as a dead man, chanting *Libera me, Domine*, in such wise that the sick man is covered with a black cloth. And the mass celebrated at his seclusion may be chosen either by the priest or by the sick man, but it is customary to say the following ...

When leaving the church after mass the priest ought to stand at the door to sprinkle him with holy water. And he ought to commend him to the care of the people. Before mass the sick man ought to make his confession in the church,

[1] Translated in Clay, R. M. (1966) pp. 273–276 from *Manuale ad Usum Insignis Ecclesiae Sarum*; translation reprinted here by permission of Frank Cass & Co. Ltd.

and never again; and in leading him forth the priest again begins the responsorium *Libera me*, *Domine*, with the other versicles. Then when he has come into the open fields he does as is aforesaid; and he ends by imposing prohibitions upon him in the following manner:—

"I forbid you ever to enter churches, or to go into a market, or a mill, or a bakehouse, or into any assemblies of people.

I forbid you ever to wash your hands or even any of your belongings in spring or stream of water of any kind; and if you are thirsty you must drink water from your cup or some other vessel.

I forbid you ever henceforth to go out without your leper's dress, that you may be recognized by others; and you must not go outside your house unshod.

I forbid you, wherever you may be, to touch anything which you wish to buy, otherwise than with a rod or staff to show what you want.

I forbid you ever henceforth to enter taverns or other houses if you wish to buy wine; and take care even that what they give you they put into your cup.

I forbid you to have intercourse with any woman except your own wife.

I command you when you are on a journey not to return an answer to any one who questions you, till you have gone off the road to leeward, so that he may take no harm from you; and that you never go through a narrow lane lest you should meet some one.

I charge you if need require you to pass over some toll-way through rough ground, or elsewhere, that you touch no posts or things whereby you cross, till you have first put on your gloves.

I forbid you to touch infants or young folk, whosoever they may be, or to give to them or to others any of your possessions.

I forbid you henceforth to eat or drink in any company except that of lepers. And know that when you die you will be buried in your own house, unless it be, by favour obtained beforehand, in the church."

And note that before he enters his house, he ought to have a coat and shoes of fur, his own plain shoes, and his signal the clappers, a hood and a cloak, two pairs of sheets, a cup, a funnel, a girdle, a small knife, and a plate. His house ought to be small, with a well, a couch furnished with coverlets, a pillow, a chest, a table, a seat, a candlestick, a shovel, a pot, and other needful articles.

When all is complete the priest must point out to him the ten rules which he has made for him; and let him live on earth in peace with his neighbour. Next must be pointed out to him the ten commandments of God, that he may live in heaven with the saints, and the priest repeats them to him in the presence of the people. And let the priest also point out to him that every day each faithful christian is bound to say devoutly *Pater Noster*, *Ave Maria*, *Credo in Deum*, and *Credo in Spiritum*, and to protect himself with the sign of the cross, saying often *Benedicite*. When the priest leaves him he says: "Worship God and give thanks to God. Have patience, and the Lord will be with thee. Amen."

2. Constitutiones Hospitalis domus leprosorum de Shirburne—

Regulations of Sherburn leper hospital (founded 1181), confirmed by Richard Kellawe, bishop of Durham (1311–16)[1].

These are the regulations of the leper hospital at Sherburn.

First, the said Bishop Hugo laid down in the chapel of the said house, there be always three priests and four clerks to serve at the altars of God and St. Mary Magdalene and St. Nicholas; two of these are to serve at the altar of St. Mary Magdalene on a weekly basis, one to celebrate chanting appropriate to the season and the other the weekly offices for the faithful, time and time about; the third priest is to officiate at the altar of St. Nicholas and always say mass for the dead, and this mass is also for the leper sisters[2] below whose house, on the south side, the chapel is situated.

In his time the said Bishop Richard of Durham added a fourth chaplain to whom he assigned the office of the blessed Virgin Mary in a new chapel which he built in her honour on the north side of the main chapel; there the fourth priest is to celebrate with solemnity a mass to the blessed Virgin Mary which is to be for the leper brothers[3] and will be the last celebration each day, for the benefit both of the brothers too weak or ill to arise early and of the priests who, their own duties completed, will all take part. On Sunday and major festivals the last mass will be a great one in the main chapel in which all the priests and clerks will take part; on those days the doors will be open for sisters and brothers alike so that all can meet in the brothers' chapel, entering and leaving in silence, the brothers preceded by their prior and the sisters followed by their prioress; at the end of the mass the sisters will return to their own house and their door will be shut.

Hugo also laid down that a master of the house should be appointed—a priest if the right man can be found but a layman if a better man is available. He is to provide the priests with all they need for their duties, to celebrate mass himself when and where he chooses, and to carry out his duties in so modest a way as not to keep more than three horses unless strictly necessary. To serve and assist the priests three clerks were allocated (or four if the master is not a priest) who are to help the priests in their sacred offices, and of whom at least one is to be a deacon.

All the priests and clerks are to sleep in a room next to the chapel, except for one whom the Master may wish to have with him in his room, and all are to lunch and dine with the master in the hall unless necessity dictates otherwise.

The same Bishop Richard also laid down that the priests are to get up in the middle of the night in the winter to complete their night offices and when these

[1] Hutchinson (1787), pp. 601-605.

[2] *sororum leprosarum.*

[3] *fratrum leprosorum.*

are finished sleep until morning. They will then return to the church in silence and after ringing the bell for the appropriate hour, chant the divine offices for that particular time. In summer they are to arise at such a time that the night office be completed at dawn and they should then stay where they are before resuming the divine offices in the prescribed manner.

Richard also ordained that there should always be a flame in the great chapel in the presence of the Lord's body and blood, and that at any celebration of any high mass in the great chapel, or mass to the blessed Virgin Mary, two candles at least should be lighted.

The same bishop also laid down that according to the statutes of his predecessor Hugo of Durham five groups of lepers, or sixty five persons in all, should always live there and be fed and clothed from the resources of the house. Every brother and sister is to have one loaf per day weighing five marks and one gallon of beer served so that each of them has a gallon a day. They are also to eat meat three days a week and fish four days a week; one dish whether of meat, fish, cheese, or butter will easily suffice for two people. He provided also that on major festivals during the year there be two dishes—that is, on the four days of Christmas, the Circumcision, Epiphany, the Purification, St. Cuthbert's day, Quadragesima (when fresh salmon are normally to be given for one dish if available, and failing that another fresh fish if possible), the Annunciation, St. Michael's day (when geese are to be provided for a dish, four people sharing one goose—except when the day falls on a Friday or Saturday when they are provided the next Sunday), All Saints day, etc.

As for clothing, it was laid down that each of them have every year three ells of woollen cloth white or rust-coloured, six ells of linen cloth and six ells of canvas for making towels for general use. At All Saints they are to have four trusses of straw and four at Christmas with four logs for four fires; at Easter four trusses of straw, at Pentecost four bundles of reeds, as well as four on St. John the Baptist's day and the festival of St. Mary Magdalene. When they have fresh meat or fish or eggs they are to have one measure of salt containing a twentieth part of a raser[4]. When they have no meat they are to have a raser of corn to make a cake.

When one dies what he brought with him from home should be left to the house; and in his place another is to be admitted from the same diocese if there are that many lepers there, or otherwise from elsewhere, for God is no respecter of persons.

The brothers are to elect a prior from their own members by general agreement and the sisters a prioress who under the master should look after them conscientiously.

The regulation of the lepers is like this: the leper brothers are to remain by themselves, and likewise the sisters by themselves, where they are to have four fires for which every day from St. Michael's to All Saints' they receive two baskets of peat. ... At Christmas they are to have four large tree-trunks for the four fires, each one large enough for a cart to itself. In summer when the peat is cut they are to have the broken fragments of the other peat.

If any brother or sister leper is so sick that hope is lost, he should have a fire, a candle and all he needs until he recovers or dies. Then on the day when anyone is buried drink and food should be given to the burial party. Likewise on the day he cuts their clothes, their tailor should be given food and drink. Every Sunday they are to receive ten white loaves, that is five for the brothers and five for the

[4] *rasarii*: 3 rasers = 1 quarter.

sisters, to be given at the discretion of the prior and prioress to those who are weakest. It is to be made clear also that they are to receive at least once or twice every week of the year fresh fish when available, or failing fresh fish red herrings, cheese or butter according to the season; when they do get herring, three each; when butter or cheese, a weight of one and a half stones for all of them together. From Easter to Pentecost in default of fish, butter or cheese they should have eggs from time to time, three each; from Pentecost until St. Michael's they are not to be given red herring and particular care must be taken that nothing bad, mouldy or rotten is issued. At Quadragesima they are to have two rasers of beans for roasting; on St. Michael's day two rasers of apples. Next they should have a kitchen and a cook to prepare their food, also a fire adequate for cooking and appropriate utensils: one lead cistern and two earthenware pots, one table, one wine vessel, one bowl and two basins to take their beer and one for washing; in the house itself they should have four lead cisterns, four pans, four tripods, two tubs, and one spade for burying the dead. Then they should sometimes grow greens, sometimes leeks, sometimes beans, according to the season. ... On days when they have fish they should be given for cooking them one measure of salt containing a sixty-third part of a raser to salt the sauce. The old woman who ministers to the sick should have each week three loaves of bread and one dish of meat or fish according to the season.

They are to have two washerwomen who should before all other work on Saturdays wash the lepers heads; they should wash their clothes twice a week and their utensils every day.

They are to have one chaplain from the above-mentioned four priests, assigned to holy duties, hearing confessions and everything appropriate to fulfilment of his sacred task, and reading the gospel in the houses of the lepers on Sundays and other major feasts, for those sick who cannot go to church. He is likewise to perform the funerals for the dead.

Leave is given for their common or particular servants[5] to come and go without hindrance, sell what is not required, buy what is required, and carry out other business. Leave is also given for their friends and well-wishers to visit and comfort them without hindrance and stay with them overnight if they have come a long way and are rare visitors; but those they know well and live nearby should return home the same day.

All are to work together for the house and allow no harm to come to it; their water supply is to be looked after so that they allow no interruption to it, and they should be allowed to come and go without hindrance to the spring near the cemetery where they obtain water for washing the house.

The doors should not be closed before the ringing of the curfew.

They are to have a bier for carrying the dead.

To encourage their observance, they should be given a stick which their prior should look after in the manner of a schoolmaster, with which he is to correct the disobedient and those who break the rules, and to encourage the faithless and negligent.

But if anyone is disobedient and difficult and refuses to be corrected by the stick he is to be deprived of all but bread and water once, twice, three times; if he still persists in his disobedience and willfulness he is to be expelled from

[5] It is not clear whether the particular servants, *servientes speciales*, were servants with special tasks or personal servants.

the community of the brothers and someone else immediately admitted in his place.

When any brother or sister dies, they are all to say for him in the next thirty days 300 Our Fathers apart from the usual daily prayers.

The master is to audit the house accounts four times a year, that is in the four quarters of the year, with his servants.

The brothers and sisters are to receive every year five shillings and five pence on the day of the raising of the holy cross, the anniversary of Martin of the Holy Cross one-time master of the house.

All this Richard by the grace of God bishop of Durham laid down and confirmed in his writing and instructed to be observed without fail.

3. Statuta Hospitalis de Sancto Juliano—

Regulations of the leper hospital of St. Julian near St. Albans (founded 1146)—revised by Abbot Michael in 1344[1]

Michael, by divine leave abbot of the monastery of St. Albans, of the order of St. Benedict and of the diocese of Lincoln to our beloved sons in Christ, the master and brothers of the hospital of St. Julian near St. Albans, in our jurisdiction and patronage, greetings with the Saviour's blessing and our own: the following is to be observed unfailingly for ever. Care for the task committed to us, and exercise of our judgment, prompt us to ensure provision with all possible foresight for those things which lead to an increase in our worship of God, and to restore as best we can to the path of certainty those things which the pious devotion of our predecessors ordained (praiseworthily to be sure but perhaps with too little certainty). Our predecessor Gaufred of happy memory with the approval of his whole convent, gathered together the lazars[2] to the church of St. Julian near St. Albans, now generally known as the hospital of St. Julian. For their support he gave to the monastery—the monks and the servants—the task of protecting them and praying for the souls of King Offa and others. He collected much goods for this task of support which our predecessor and his convent took upon themselves, and we too are obliged to his benefactors, whom we might more accurately call our benefactors. He also assigned an equal part to a single priest whose task was to minister the church's sacraments to these same lepers[3]; and in the charter of that time more provisions are made. But he omitted to lay down a definite number of lazars, to make regulations about divine service, and to give instructions as to how and by whom their wealth should be controlled, for they themselves cannot control these things because of their bodily infection; and for this latter reason there were often many fewer lepers in the hospital than could adequately have been sustained by its income.

For example there were sometimes only one or two, and only when there were three was it a proper community: also in certain times of decline there was less worthy service to God, while the gifts, which were too much for these one, two or three lepers, were diverted to unworthy and damnable uses and were embezzled by usurpers in whose possession they remain even now; thus resources have been lost. For these reasons we have had the following rules drawn up and assembled in full maturity: to increase the worship of God; to drive out this harmful uncertainty by providing definite and provident regulations; to set out the arrangement and organisation of the hospital, which experience itself will prove useful; from a deep desire for the glory and honour of our Lord Jesus Christ, His blessed

[1] Matthew Paris (1684), *Auctarium Additamentorum* pp. 1159-1171.

[2] *lazaros.*

[3] *leprosis.*

mother Mary, St. Alban, St. Julian and all God's saints, and for the souls of King Offa and all the hospital's benefactors; and for the satisfaction of the monastery, the monks, the brothers and the servants as they carry out those duties which we are obliged to our benefactors for enabling us to fulfil.

First of all we consider that the resources of the hospital have by the generosity of the faithful been so substantially increased since its foundation and first endowment that there are hardly enough lepers to be found who are prepared to come to the hospital and lead a life bound by its regulations, and to occupy the hospital to the full capacity of its facilities. More than three lepers and also some priests can live together on the income of the hospital for the greater glorification of God. To these priests we can transfer some of our responsibilities, obligations for which purpose the hospital was founded, for we ourselves are obliged to celebrate divine service for our benefactors. After deliberation with our convent and taking account of our own previous ideas we decree and lay down that by our ordinance there shall always be six lepers in the hospital, living apart from the healthy because of the risk of contagion. We also decree that all the statutes and rules must be strictly observed, and they are to live as formerly under the ancient regulations set out below. We further desire and command that they be looked after in the traditional way from the resources of the hospital. We have had all this set out to avoid any scruple of doubt.

The admission of leper brothers

Because the organisation of the said hospital in both spiritual and temporal matters is our absolute responsibility, and the brothers in the hospital are customarily received and admitted in our name by the abbot of the said monastery, whoever he may be at the time, or by the abbot's archdeacon, we give these instructions for the future. As far as the admission of leper brothers is concerned, we wish preference to be given to monks of the said monastery; to our own kindred, especially to those who have connections with the monks, who have been afflicted with the signs of leprosy; and to those who came from the town of St. Albans and elsewhere in our jurisdiction. They are to be received according to the rules written here provided nothing in the following debars them.

The admission of brothers and their vows

Those who by permission of the lord abbot enter the hospital (without his permission none may enter) are absolved. Any married man who has to enter should make a solemn vow of chastity, both himself and his wife before the lord archdeacon, as ordinary of the place, and before the brothers of the house. If after admission he incontinently breaks his vow he should be expelled according to the custom of the house, and should be returned to his wife, if she be alive, and discharge his conjugal debts to her. Similarly if his wife goes against her vow she should be similarly punished. But if she should fall into misfortune then her husband should be punished as though he were guilty of incontinence.

No married lepers to be received amongst the brothers in the hospital

Since man and wife are made one flesh in married union and it is not possible for one part to turn to the Lord and the other to remain in the world, we follow the sacred canons in prohibiting any married leper from ever being admitted as a brother to the hospital unless his wife either takes to the religious life, or else is of such an age that she can remain in the world without suspicion of incontinence and has made a vow of perpetual chastity. Moreover, whether it is the man or his wife who happens to become a leper, if the sick one demands payment from his or her body then, according to the general teaching of the apostle, what is due must be paid.

The mode of admission to the hospital
The brothers who are admitted to the hospital are to be on probation until they make their vows. During this time more can be learned of their morals and conversation through their behaviour and activity. During their probation period they will not be admitted as equals to the councils of the brothers in their chapters.

Concerning the professions of the brothers of St. Julian
I brother N. promise and by the sacrament of the body standing before the holy gospels affirm before God and all the saints in this church built in honour of St. Julian the confessor, in the presence of the lord archdeacon N., that all the days of my life I shall depend on and obey the precepts of the lord abbot of St. Albans, whoever he be at the time, and his archdeacon; in nothing shall I disobey unless any orders are given which are contrary to God's will. I shall never steal, nor make a false accusation against any brother, nor lay violent hands on a brother. I shall not break my vow of chastity. Without leave from the brothers I shall not make any changes in things to be acquired or others to be left as a bequest. I shall studiously avoid all kinds of usury as monstrous and hateful to God. I shall never plan, help or act in word or deed, in such a way, myself or through someone else, that any custodian or master be set over the lepers of St. Julian other than he whom the lord abbot of St. Albans has chosen to appoint. I shall be satisfied without complaint or murmur with the food and drink and other things given and offered to me by the master according to the use and custom of the house. I shall not transgress the bounds laid down or the special instructions of my superiors without their consent. If I am found to have transgressed any rule noted above I am ready and willing that the lord abbot or his substitute should punish me according to the type and extent of my shortcomings just as seems best to him, and should even expel me from the congregation of brothers like an apostate without hope of return, other than by the special favour of the lord abbot.

Articles to be observed by the professed brothers of the house of St. Julian near St. Albans
Since amongst all infirmities the disease of leprosy is held in contempt, those who are struck down with such a disease ought to show themselves only at special times and places, and in their manner and their dress more contemptible and humble than other men. As the Lord says in Leviticus 'Whosoever is disfigured with leprosy should wear his clothes open, his head bare, his mouth covered with a cloth and call out that he is unclean and contaminated; and when he is leprous and unclean he is to dwell alone without the camp.' Nor should they despair or murmur against God because of this, but rather praise and glorify Him, who when He was led to His death wished to be compared to the lepers. As witness of this consider the prophet Isaiah who said 'And we thought him struck down as a leper by God, and humiliated' and recall also the memory of the blessed Job who, when

he was struck down with leprosy so badly that he was affected from the soles of his feet to the top of his head, nevertheless said nothing foolish against God.

The dress of the leper brothers

Because the hospital of St. Julian beside the wood of Eywood was founded by the abbot and convent of St. Albans especially for the lepers, and is maintained by their pious collection of alms, and because the organisation of it in both spiritual and temporal matters is known to belong to that same abbot as patron and ordinary, we with paternal solicitude considering the reputation of the hospital and its worth in God's sight desire that the brothers living there should wear such clothes as is appropriate to their infirmity.

The brothers are to have a tunic and upper tunic of russet, with a hood cut from the same, so that the sleeves of the tunic be closed as far as the hand, but not laced with knots or thread after the secular fashion. They are to wear the upper tunic closed down to the ankles, and a close cape of black cloth of the same length as the hood, as they have been accustomed of old.

The testaments of the leper brothers

We allow the leper brothers freely to bequeathe, if they wish, up to one third of the moveable possessions that they may have brought with them to the hospital or have had sent in: this third part they may leave in their last will or testament to their servants and others who have deserved well of them. The other two parts and any other goods received from the hospital or elsewhere are to remain in the hospital, to be used for the benefit of the sick brothers at the discretion of the master. If these two parts together with the other goods are altogether of so little worth as to be manifestly of little use to the sick brothers, then the master should not fail to hand them over for the use of the poor and needy. So that the division of the goods may be made efficiently and without fraud, we have laid down that each leper brother on his admission is to make an accurate inventory of all his moveable goods, with three copies—one to be lodged with our archdeacon, one with the master and the third to remain with the brother being admitted.

Instructions concerning the form of the testament

When a leper brother wishes to make his testament or to leave the third part of his goods in his last will, as described above, he is to testify or, as far as he is able, to express his wishes in the presence of the master or (if the master is busy or absent and unable to oblige) in the presence of his locum tenens, and make over the residual part of his inventory to the master or his locum. The master or his locum are to ensure that the testament or last will is written down and that the appropriate part of the inventory is set out in writing; he is to sign it with his seal and after the brother's death have the document sent to the archdeacon or his locum tenens without delay, so that by the archdeacon's authority the testament or will may be made available for the proper execution of the previously described third part. The archdeacon or his locum must hasten to do his part whatever the difficulties, so that the testament or will may be quickly executed. If the brother recovers, the document is to be returned to him. If the leper brother leaves or gives anything to anyone beyond the third part, we desire that such bequest or gift be invalid, while the disposal of the third part is none the less to stand firm.

The testaments of priestly brothers
If the priest brothers wish to make a testament or to leave anything in their will, they are carefully and correctly to follow the same rule and method, both as to the inventory and to every single other item contained in the headings above concerning testaments of lepers and the way of making a testament, under pain of the penalties clearly laid down there.

The arrangement of services
In the morning when the bell is rung for the canonical hours to be heard, all are to arise and putting on their closed capes to go to the church and hear divine service. When they have entered the church they are all to sit in order according to the time they were admitted to the hospital. No one is to presume through pride to take for himself the seat of another, unless fairness requires that the master promote someone above the rest by reason of his reverence or the dignity of his bearing and station. This early service is so to be arranged that it is not onerous to anyone, but suits the convenience of all the infirm: thus none can excuse himself, unless he be prevented by serious infirmity. So with everybody gathered together in the church, as we have said, they are to keep silence until the service is over.

The commons of the leper brothers
Let every leprous brother receive from the property of the hospital, for his living and all necessaries, whatever he has been accustomed to receive by the custom observed of old in the said hospital: namely, every week seven loaves, of which five shall be white and two brown, made from the grain as threshed from the ear; also, every seventh week, fourteen gallons of beer, or eightpence for the same. Let him have, in addition to this, on the feasts of all the saints, on the feast of St. Julian, the purification of the blessed Mary, the Annunciation, the Trinity, St. Albans, St. John the Baptist, the Assumption of the blessed Mary, and the Nativity of the same, for each feast one loaf, one jar of beer, or a penny for the same, and one obolus, which is called the charity of the aforesaid hospital; also, let every leprous brother receive, at the feast of Christmas, forty gallons of good beer, or forty pence for the same. Let each also receive on the said feast his share of two quarters of pure and clean corn, which is called the great charity. At the feast of St. Martin, each leper shall have one pig from the common stall and so that there may be a fair division of the pigs amongst the brothers, according to the custom observed of old, we desire that the pigs, according to the number of the lepers, may be brought forward in their presence if it can conveniently be done, otherwise in another place fit for the purpose; there each, according to the priority of entering the hospital, shall choose one pig (otherwise a sum of money to be distributed equal to the value of the pigs). Each leper shall receive on the feast of St. Valentine one quarter of oats for the whole of the ensuing year, and about the feast of St. John Baptist two bushels of salt, or the current price. At the feast of St. Julian and at the feast of St. Alban, one penny for the accustomed pittance, and at Easter one penny, known as "Flavvonespeni"; on Ascension day one obolus for buying potherbs. On each Wednesday in Lent they shall receive bolted corn of the weight of one of their loaves and on the feast of St. John the Baptist four shillings for clothes. At Christmas, let fourteen shillings be distributed in equal portions among the leprous brothers for their fuel through the

year, as has been ordained of old for the sake of peace and concord. Also, since, by the bounty of our Lord the King, thirty shillings and fivepence have been assigned for ever for the use of the lepers, which sum the Viscount of Hertford has to pay them annually at the feasts of Easter and Michaelmas, we command that the said 30s. and 5d. be equally divided among them in the usual manner. We desire the brothers to be contented with the aforesaid distributions, which have been accustomed to be made amongst the leprous brothers of old. The residue of the property of the said hospital, we order and decree to be applied to the support of the master and priests of the said hospital.

The entrance of women

Because through the entry of women scandals and immodest evils often arise, we most strictly forbid that any woman should enter the brothers' hospice excepting only the general housekeeper, who should be of mature years and good conversation and concerning whom there could be no breath of suspicion. Nor should she venture into their houses at suspicious times, but at proper hours so that her coming and going may be seen by all. However, if a mother, sister or other honest matron should come there to visit the sick, she is to have access to the one with whom she wishes to talk by permission of the custodian of the house; in no other circumstances is any woman to enter. Women of easy fame and low reputation are under no conditions to enter the hospital.

Eating with women

No brother is to be allowed to invite women apart from those mentioned above to eat with him in his house for the reasons just stated. This will be with the special permission of the master, provided that no woman stays with them beyond the proper hour but withdraws at the agreed time. Any one who does otherwise will be punished as though guilty of unchastity.

Concerning loitering

None of the brothers is to venture beyond the bounds of his hospice towards the royal road, except with his cape closed and on his way to or from the church. Nor are they to loiter or wander in the said street before or after the service, or at any hour of the day before or after dinner. But when the divine service is over they are to enter their hospice with all speed, except when anyone wishes to stay behind in the church to be free for prayer.

More concerning loitering

We also forbid loitering on the path which extends along in front of the brothers' houses towards the royal road; no brother is to converse there with another. If any of the brothers wishes to talk with another he is to cross the path quickly to the other side without loitering, and enjoy his conversation, except when someone from outside meets him by chance, in which case he can speak with him briefly and pass over. But if any upright and honest man comes there to visit a sick brother he is to come in to him and they are to converse about what is good.

The custodian under the master

None of the brothers is under any circumstances to venture to the mill or the brewery, except the one who is given this responsibility. When he enters he is not to go near the bread or the beer, touching or handling it in any way, because it is not right for men with this disease to handle what is destined for the common use of men.

Concerning locking up

The gates which open on to the garden are to be kept shut and guarded on account of the scandals and other evils which could arise from free entry through them. No brother is to go out through them for longer than a minute or when someone needs relief by reason of particular infirmity (when a superior will give special permission). As for the gates towards the square on one side and the royal road on the other side, nobody is to go out through these except for the one who is given the task of agriculture; he will go out from time to time to supervise the carters and the sowers to see if they are working faithfully and carefully.

Leper brothers not to venture away without permission

Those who are afflicted with leprosy are by general custom separated from communion with other men, and in God's law it is generally laid down that lepers should be placed 'outside the camp'. As a rule we have therefore laid down that the leper brothers shall never leave the closed interior of the hospital, or its outer boundaries laid down of old without permission of the master. The master is not to give his permission unless the reason given him is such that by its merits it deserves to persuade and move him to grant it. We do, however, grant full authority to the master to give permission for a leper brother to go to the town of St. Albans, or to venture through the middle of the town to a place up to a mile from the hospital, or to spend a night away from the hospital, or to go to the well, the mill or the grange.

Permission of the archdeacon for going beyond the boundaries

No brother is to venture beyond the normal agreed boundaries in order to wander or travel through the countryside. If anyone does, he is to be punished by being deprived of his liberty. Anyone who absents himself from his house for a whole day and night without special permission from the lord abbot or his archdeacon will be treated as a fugitive and will not be allowed back, except by favour and permission of the lord abbot.

Concerning discord amongst the brothers

The brothers should listen to each other and show each other respect, as the Apostle said, "outstripping each other in mutual esteem". If anyone is found contentious and to be sowing discord amongst the brothers he is to be reproached on the first two occasions; if he does not mend his ways he is to be punished by deprivation of his liberty until his behaviour is completely satisfactory.

Concerning the making of agreements

If at any time the brothers wish for the common good to discuss the management of the house they are to enter the church and, after excluding all lay people and unprofessed brothers (since they ought not to be concerned in the common council), are to discuss amongst themselves what is best and consistent with the plans and desires of the master. But private and false agreements which ought rather to be termed conspiracies or plots, we absolutely forbid and declare void.

Punishment for disobedience

The articles above we instruct to be kept without fail. If anyone contravenes them in any way and holds their observance in contempt he is to be punished by loss of his freedom, or some other punishment chosen by the master is to be inflicted on him; the severity of the punishment should correspond to the quality and quantity of guilt.

Regulations concerning the reading of the regulations

Lest the leper brothers and priests be able to excuse themselves from observance of the ordinances under the pretext of ignorance, we decree and command that the regulations we have ordained, in so far as they concern the leper brothers or affect the chapel brothers, should on four separate occasions each year be read and explained clearly and openly, and in the vulgar tongue, so that each of them may be able to understand plainly what he ought to observe and how.

For the perpetual maintenance of the ordinances, and in witness of them, we have placed our seal upon them in our above-mentioned monastery on the 11th February AD 1344.

4. Ordinacio Hospitalis Enicopensis—

Regulations of the Enköping leper hospital, Sweden, given by Archbishop Birger of Uppsala (1367-83)[1]

In the name of our Lord Jesus Christ and the glorious virgin Mary His mother.

Those who have been admitted to the hospital of Enköping or who will be admitted in the future, those poor are yet heirs of God and co-heirs with Christ. Despising worldly things and dedicating themselves and their possessions to Christ they must ardently and freely devote themselves to vigils, fasting, prayers and other services, and to the praises of God. Their comings, goings and prayers must be acceptable to God. To this end we Birger, by divine mercy archbishop of Uppsala, have prepared and laid down the following statutes and rules to be observed most carefully by the inmates and the staff for all time.

First, men and women afflicted with leprosy[2] must be carefully sought out and found by the warden of the hospital throughout the diocese of Uppsala: if they are poor they must be admitted to the hospital without charge. Those who have moveable possessions are to be admitted with their possessions, which are to be used for the common good under the warden's supervision; they, or their heirs, can be compelled if they resist. As far as immoveable assets are concerned the same usage applies as is normally followed by the laws and practices of the country relating to other goods given or bequeathed to churches and other holy places.

Next, we wish the following rules to be observed in the hospital, each of them is to receive every day two pure barley loaves and at special festivals—Christmas, the Circumcision, Epiphany, the Purification, Easter, the Ascension, Corpus Christi, St. John the Baptist, the Assumption, St. Michael's day, All Saints' day and St. Nicholas' day—each is to have two barley loaves and one wheaten loaf. On each of those days they are also to share half a jar[3] of good beer if there are ten of them, or a whole jar if they number between twelve and twenty. But every day in Lent each is to have one barley loaf, one wheaten loaf and two herring, likewise on fast days other than in Lent. Also in Lent the community as a whole is to be given fifty cod and fifty dried pike, a bushel of peas and two smoked salmon. If herring cannot be obtained outside Lent then the prescribed portion—that is, two herring—are to be supplied by the warden in the form of dried and fresh fish. If there are eight inmates[4] they are also to have the following (if there are more than this, or some are so weak as to need more, these portions are to be increased according to the judgement of the management): first, every week except

[1] Ehlers (1898), pp. 69–74.

[2] *morbus leprae.*

[3] *lagena.*

[4] *pauperes*: it is clear both from the instruction to search out lepers and from the later note of danger of infection that the inmates were not just paupers; the idiom was probably "Christ's poor".

in Lent each person is to have one mark of butter; next, they are to share half a talent of lard and one and a half talents of smoked beef if there are ten persons; if there are more, then amounts should be increased according to numbers and need.

These weekly rations are to be given to them even if a saint's day or other church fast happens to occur. On every fourth week day in summer, unless it be a fast, they are to share an urn of soured milk and on Sunday an urn of fresh milk. Every week they are to have one jar of beer for between five and eight people, but a half jar for only four; if there are between ten and fifteen, one and a half jars, and two jars if there are between sixteen and twenty. This beer should not be freshly brewed but should be seven days old; the jar should be full. If there are eight people they are to have about Martinmas every year two tuns of grain and two talents of fat for candles. Every year about Michaelmas every eight persons are to share three pounds of salt, about Easter two pounds, and about St. John the Baptist's day one pound.

Every year at about Martinmas each person is to have eight ells[5] of cloth from the hospital. At Christmas and on St. John the Baptist's day, everyone is to be given a pair of shoes. At All Saints the management is to give the house servant for his services half a mark of money, and the same again before Easter.

Further, we desire and declare that the utensils needed for the inmates be given to them by the warden, namely one cauldron of five urns capacity, one cauldron of one urn capacity, one pot of one urn capacity, one jar and two urn measures, unless the number of people or usage require more. When these utensils are worn out or broken they are to be replaced by the warden.

As for the keeping of fast days by the sick we have ordained that those who have reached years of discretion should one and all (unless afflicted by such serious sickness that they cannot fast without danger to their life) be bound to take part together in fasts according to the statutes of the church and the customs of the land; if fresh fish and other foods are in very short supply in Lent we give our permission for milk foods on alternate days until the middle of Lent, but from then until Easter day they ought to abstain from such things—a matter which we leave to their consciences to decide.

We have also laid down that no one, however powerful and from whatever condition or class he comes, once he has dedicated himself to God in the hospital is to venture to leave the gates of the hospital for churches, meetings, or any other gatherings whatsoever, that is if he does not wish to lose the rations due to him for the following week, and wants to avoid even worse punishment if he persists in disobedience. If this instruction is disobeyed the christian population is likely to become infected by conversation and contact with the hospital patients. But for the begging of alms, mazers should be placed around the chapel or elsewhere in their church-yard where there are bystanders and at other times, so that they may receive more alms from passers-by or visitors.

People of both sexes living in the hospital who are strong enough and able to work ought to help and work together with their own hands in summer and autumn to bring in the hay and to harvest the grain in wagons to the granary.

As for legacies to the hospital itself and things left or intended to be left to individuals there, we wish the following to be observed: if they come to the hospital in the form of ready money, gold or silver, they are to be spent in the decoration

[5] 1 ell = 2 feet.

or structure of the chapel; while if, whatever their size, legacies of this kind are left to individuals in the hospital, they are to be given to those individuals, less a small proportion. But if the means of life are bequeathed, for instance cattle, pigs, sheep, flour, wheat, or other things which are necessary for the feeding or clothing of the inmates, then they should divide and dispose these things equally amongst themselves. In the event of bequests of horses, domestic oxen or other animals useful for work they should be handed over according to the instructions of the warden for the use of the hospital. If special items of food are bequeathed the warden is to take these for hospital use and give them to those in most need.

It must be noted that the warden is to have this statute read without fail in the presence of the whole community of the place once a year, that is on the day after Martinmas. The warden or superintendent of the house will also be bound to make or render every year to us or our successors a proper and careful account of the administration and expenses of the house for which he has been responsible, and a statement of when and where it can be seen.

5. Regulations of the leper hospital of St. Mary Magdalene, Exeter, as restated early in the fifteenth century[1]

The mayor, bailiffs, and twenty-four common council, are to chuse yearly a governor or warden, who, by himself or his sufficient deputy, shall govern and rule the impotent and sick persons within the said hospital, according to the orders and ordinances of the said house, which are as followeth:—

First—That any brother and sister admitted and being one of the company of the said house, shall daily twice upon every day at least, unless he or she be sick and not able to come to the chappel, and then and there to hear such divine service as shall be said before them, upon pain that every one failing, unless he or she be sick or have some reasonable cause of absence, to fast with bread and water for three days together.

Also no brother nor sister shall go or pass out of that house beyond the bryde, without the gate of the said hospital, without the licence of the warden or his deputy, upon pain to be put into the stocks and to have but bread and water for one day.

No brother shall enter into the house or lodging of any sister, nor any sister to enter into the house of any sister (brother ?) without special licence of the warden or his deputy, upon pain to be punished in the stocks or otherwise, at the discretion of the warden.

No brother shall belie his sister, nor sister shall belie any of her brothers, nor yet any of them shall belie the warden or his deputy, upon pain to have but bread and water and to sit in the stocks for three days.

If any brother or sister do in any malice or displeasure, in the presence of any person, call one the other of them thief, or any evil name, or do revile one the other, shall likewise be in the stocks and fast with bread and water for three days.

If any brother or sister do maliciously, slanderously, and in displeasure, revile the master, warden, or his deputy he shall fast with bread and water and lie in the stocks twelve days.

If any brother or sister do in anger, malice, or displeasure, strike or lay violent hands upon one the other, he shall be punished in the stocks, and have but bread and water for thirty days.

If any brother or sister do disclose, utter, or betray any of the secrets of their house, or of the warden or his deputy, and thereof by due proof be convicted, he shall be punished in the stocks, and have but bread and water for twelve days.

No brother nor sister shall receive nor lodge into his house any stranger or other person whatsoever, without licence of the warden or his deputy.

That no guest being received or lying in the house shall lie with his wife, nor

[1] Shapter (1835), pp. 30–33.

any wife with her husband within the precinct of the said hospital, in one and the same bed.

If any brother or sister do threaten the other of life or limb, shall abide the same pain and punishment as if he smite or hurt him.

If any brother or sister do pick or steal from the other, shall be punished as if he had gone out of the doors beyond the place appointed, and as by the warden shall be thought good. Anno 30. Hen. IV. Martin Roff.

6. Ældre Svendborg-Dokument 1486—

Regulations for St. George's hospital, Svendborg, Denmark, in 1486[1]

We Karl, by God's grace bishop in Odense, Gregorius Marsvin, our dear gracious lord's provost in Nyborg, Hanns Andersen, mayor of Svendborg, Niels Mogensen, Hendrich Jensen, Peder Ebsen, Røyter Persen, Oluf Andersen, Madz ... and Marten Verchmester, councillors and citizens in the latter town declare that according to the command of our dear gracious lord we were gathered in the council hall in Svendborg on the Friday after St. Ambrosius day in 1486. ...

The manorial dues and interests annually granted the warden and the servants belonging to St. George's hospital[2] in corn, butter, money, lambs, geese, hens and pannage, or whatever it may be, are to be shared equally between the sick brothers and sisters and the eight healthy brothers and sisters, who should nurse and work for their living. Likewise their priest is to receive annually 5 marks for three masses which he must say for them each week in the church; if he also wants a share of the income of the hospital with the brothers and sisters, then he may have it because he is their parish priest and has to give them their sacrament; in that event he must be formerly admitted to the hospital like any other brother or sister.

Now if any of the eight healthy brothers and sisters, who have to go out and beg alms on behalf of the others, are married and husband or wife happens to die, the spouse should never marry again or in any way live an unseemly life, but should live a pure life after the fashion of a monk or nun. If husband or wife of one of the sick should happen to die the spouse should not marry again but should devote himself or herself to the sick. Their proctor[3] should be elected by all the brothers and sisters themselves, and is to receive the share of two brothers and sisters; in return he is to supply the tenants with food and beer and give them hospitality when they pay their manorial dues. He is to share out the income of the hospital in cash and kind as aforementioned.

Each tenant who has a good farm and is able must provide the proctor with two horses twice a year, and those who could not easily afford this are to provide two horses a year: they should all provide shelter, beer and forage for those begging alms on behalf of the monastery. Those tenants who do not pay liberty money[4] must give one day's work to the proctor in the rye harvest and two day's work in the barley harvest, but those who do pay are exempt; they must also help to provide a cart for him when he travels on official business.

1 Ehlers (1898), pp. 74–79.
2 *St. Jørgensgaard.*
3 *Ridesvend.*
4 *frihedspenge.*

Three locks must be placed on each church almsbox and on the safe place in which they hide their documents and charters (which must be kept in the church). The key for one lock should be kept by the warden, one by the priest and the third jointly by the churchwarden and proctor; none of the other two keyholders have the power to prevent the proctor and the churchwarden opening the box, if need be.

Alms which are put in the poor box as *frankalmoin*, table money, and that pound of corn which is sent to the church from the farm, are to be used to keep the church in good repair and decoration, but if it is not so used then the proctor and the church warden should annually present the account to the priest.

They should provide themselves with a horse and cart to gather God's alms from the good people and they should themselves provide fodder for the horses.

There are also some who are suffering from such a foul disease that they cannot remain amongst healthy people in the surrounding parishes; they should therefore allow themselves to be admitted, and if they are admitted without any endowment they should pay an admission fee, if it is within their means.

Only eight healthy brothers and sisters should live there to care for the sick and to beg alms; they should have an equal share of income and provisions with the sick. When either a sick or healthy brother or sister dies their possessions shall remain in the house[5], and their belongings shall be used by all the brothers and sisters and must not be taken away. If one of the brothers or sisters should commit a crime, the fine shall be used by the brothers and sisters in the house. If someone is sentenced to death, he shall be executed at the court of Sund hundred[6] and his possessions or fine according to the law shall be given to all the brothers and sisters.

The warden is forbidden to fell trees or to let others fell trees or spoil the woods belonging to the house; he must not permit any one to cut down trees in it without the permission of the proctor and the church warden. ...

When all these above-mentioned paragraphs had been drawn up, read and made clear to Erik Christensen, who has been appointed warden to St. George's hospital and its estates by our dear gracious lord and to Mickel Poulsen, Reimart Madsen and several brothers and sisters who had attended the meeting as representatives of all the brothers and sisters, then they all agreed and were in all respects pleased with the articles. As a further manifestation of their satisfaction with the above-mentioned we append our signatures at the bottom of this letter.

[5] *Kloster*: literally monastery; the reference is clearly to the St. Jorgensgaard, the leper hospital, which was of course a religious house.

[6] *Sundtz Herridtz Ting*.

7. Kong Hans' Anordning om Trætte mellem Forstanderen i Næstved og Lemmerne, 1492

King Hans' decree concerning the quarrel between the warden and lepers in St. George's hospital, Næstved, Denmark, in 1492[1]

We Hans, by God's grace king of Denmark, Norway the Vends and Goths, chosen king of Sweden etc. hereby declare that when we were in Næstved Jens Boesen, who is now warden at St. George's hospital[2] there, and the brothers and sisters admitted there, came before us to plead their grievances. The brothers and sisters claimed that they were unable to obtain their income from the said Jens Boesen, and mentioned other quarrels and disagreements between them. Following the council of the government of our dear Denmark we made this decree and pronouncement:—

Firstly, that the warden, or any of his successors must point out to the women-folk of the sick brothers and sisters that they shall look after them and prepare their food, keep their clothes clean with lye, and anything else that they may need. They[3] must provide them with house-keeping, firewood, and anything else they may need, together with their keep of food and beer according to the following: on the meat day with bacon, beef, cabbage and an unsalted dish, whichever is obtainable at the time of year, or another dish in its place, and in the morning porridge, fish or herring as is necessary with as much beer as is reasonable. He shall keep a chaplain who shall read three masses per week, Sunday, Wednesday and Friday, build and improve the church and the farm, maintain it and keep the servants of the monastery to the law, and in no circumstances allow the forests to be cut down. He shall also, as far as possible, improve the decoration of the church and improve it in any other way. If he is in a position to do so he shall give to the healthy brothers and sisters 11 shillings annually, one unsalted cow and one quarter of butter. From to-day no healthy brothers and sisters must be admitted, only as many sick people as are in the parish that is paying rent to the monastery; all of these should always be admitted and kept there, as it is written, and the warden can punish as he sees fit anyone who does not obey this rule.

Our mayor and council in Næstved, now and henceforth, must every month send a mayor and a councillor to stay a while in the monastery to see whether this order is kept as it is written; if there should be shortcomings then they are to inform the warden or Us.

[1] Ehlers (1898), pp. 79–80.

[2] *St. Jorgens Closter*: this again emphasises the religious nature of the house; there is no doubt that it refers to the leper hospital or *St. Jorgensgaard*.

8. Chancery warrant for proper medical examination of Joanna Nightingale of Brentwood, who refused to be isolated on suspicion of leprosy, 1468[1]

To the most Excellent . . . Edward, by the grace of God, king of England . . . We, William Hatteclyff, Roger Marshall and Dominus de Serego, doctors of Art and Medicine, your physicians and sworn to watch over the health of your person, send due reverence with humility and worship. . . .

Whereas a petition was made to you in your court of Chancery with regard to removing Joanna Nightingale of Brentwood in the county of Essex from general intercourse with mankind, because it was presumed by some of her neighbours that she was infected by foul contact of leprosy and was in fact herself a leper, upon which your writ was then prepared and afterwards directed to the sheriff of the said county in these words:—

Edward, by the grace of God, King of England and France and lord of Ireland to the sheriff of Essex, greetings. Whereas we have heard that Joanna Nightingale is a leper, and is commonly holding intercourse with the people of the aforesaid county, and mixes with them in both private and public places, and refuses to retire to a solitary place, as is customary and befitting her, to the grievous injury and, on account of the contagion of the aforesaid disease, the manifest perils of the aforesaid inhabitants: We willing to guard against such dangers, as far as in us lies, and as is just and customary in such cases, do charge you, that having taken with you certain discreet and loyal men of the county of the aforesaid Joanna, in order to obtain a better knowledge of her disease, you go to the aforesaid Joanna and cause her to be diligently viewed and examined in the presence of the aforesaid men. And if you find her to be leprous, as was recorded of her, then that you cause her to be removed in as decent a manner as possible, from all intercourse with other persons, and have her betake herself immediately to a secluded place as is the custom, lest by common intercourse of this kind injury or danger should in any wise happen to the aforesaid inhabitants. Witness my hand, at Westminster, this day of July in the eighth year of Our Reign.

Wherefore the reverend father in God, Robert, by the grace of God, lord bishop of Bath and Wells, your chancellor of England, consulted us on this subject, and determined to bring the same Joanna to us, with the intention that, according to what we have learned from our knowledge of medicine, we should give information to your highness in your Chancery, whether the said Joanna be in fact a leper or not. We, therefore wishing to obey your highness, in order that the truth on this subject might be made most plain and clear, have proceeded after this manner. First, we examined her person, and, as the older and most learned medical authors have directed in these cases, we touched and handled her and made mature, diligent and proper investigation whether the symptoms indicative of this

[1] Simpson (1842), pp. 154-155.

disease were in her or not; and after an examination and consideration of each of the points, which appeared necessary to be examined and considered, in order to arrive at a true knowledge of this doubtful matter, we found that the woman neither had been nor was a leper, nor ought, on that account to be separated from ordinary intercourse with mankind.

We are taught by medical science, that the disease of leprosy is known by many signs, also that each species of the disease, of which there are four, viz. Alopicia, Tiria, Leonina, and Elephantia, should be known and characterised by particular signs, and each should be specifically distinguished from the rest. Therefore, in the case of the woman brought before us, on going through upwards of twenty-five of the more marked signs of general leprosy we do not find that she can be proved to be leprous, by them or a sufficient number of them. And this would suffice, generally, to free her from the suspicion of leprosy, since it is not possible for any to labour under the disease in whom the greater part of these signs are not found. But, in order to give our opinion on the individual species, going through upwards of forty distinctive signs of the different varieties of leprosy, we do not find that this woman is to be marked as suffering under any of the four kinds, but is utterly free and untainted, as we have signified by word of mouth to your highness in your said Chancery, and we are prepared to declare the same more fully to your highness by scientific process, if and wherever it shall be necessary.

In testimony whereof, we, the said William Hatticlyff, Roger Marshall, and Dominus de Serego, have signed our name with our proper hands, and alternately affixed our seals.

9. Petition of Nicholas Harris, footpostman of Totnes, to the Royal College of Physicians of London for a certificate that he was not a leper, 1620[1]

To the right Worshippful the President, Censores and the rest of the learned and juditious Doctors of Phisick of that famous renouwned Colledge in the Hon: Cittie of London.

The humble petition of Nicholas Harris late footpost (for almost 40 years together) for ye towne of Totnes in Devonshire.

Right honourable & worthie Doctors

It is not unknowne to many worshippfull and others both of this honourable cittie, and also in ye countery, that I have done longe, faitefull and painifull service, in my place many yeares, to ye irresuperable decay of my aged and binumed carkaise. In regarde whereof (for my maintinance during ye rest of my irkesome life) it pleased some of that towne of Totnes (my worshipfull and worthie good friendes) to appointe me, a beinge in an Almeshouse there, which was my desired content.

But so it is right worshippfulls that I founde opposition (whether upon just cause, or ill will I know not) and the Magistrates of that towne were informed that I was an uncleane manne and a Leaper, not fitte to come or be admitted into the company of cleane persons; By meanes whereof I was, and am suspended, and put by the said place, till I could either gett my cure, or by good testymony certifie that I am not so infected and polluted; In regard whereof, I your poor petitioner have undertaken a long and tedious Journey to this honourable cittie and made my humble petition to ye right worshipfull the President, governors and chirurgions of St. Bartholomew's hospital, cravinge to be viewed, which they did accordinglie, and certified theire opinion as by the said certificate, under some of theire hands appeareth.

My humble petition and swyte is in like manner to your worshippfulls further that you will be pleased for God's sake to commiserate my distressed estate, and that I may by you againe be reviewed and likewise censured, and accordinglie either out of your Charity be apointed for my cure; or out of your goodness to certifie that I am free of the said reputed Leprosie and infection (as formerlie those worthy gentlemen have done) that I maie be relieved in that manner as my worshippfull good friendes propounded (as aforesaid) the rather for that my dwellinge is so farre from this citty, and my bodie feeble, and unable to travile hither again, if there should be any further question be made concerninge the same disease. And I shall be bound and assuredly will pray for your worshippfulls etc.

[1] See Figure 24.

3rd June 1620.[2]

Wee whose names are underwritten upon this Petition have veiwed the body of this petitioner and in our censures he is free from ye imputed diseases.

Thomas Moundeford pres. Coll. med. Lond:
John Argent
Richard Andrewes Censores
Sidney Baskerville
Matthew Gwynn Regestr.

[2] At first sight the date on the document appears to be 1626 and it was so read by Windeatt in 1880. In fact it is 1620 with the 0 caught up in a flourish on an h in the line beneath. Mr. L. M. Payne, Librarian of the Royal College of Physicians, has kindly confirmed that these signatories were in office in 1619/20 and not in 1626. Windeatt also misread several of their signatures; the names given here are those which are confirmed by the records of the college.

10. Ett af Gustaf II Adolf utfärdadt patent ...

Royal patent of Gustaf II Adolf of Sweden, July 15th, 1619, authorising the foundation of Sjählö leper hospital in Finland[1]

We Gustav... declare that because we have formed the impression that the infectious plague and disease of leprosy, which is a divine punishment for sin, is spreading and becoming common in Finland, and not least because those who are afflicted with it mix carelessly with those who are healthy and live amongst them, thus the disease must be prevented and retarded in as far as it is humanly possible. In order to separate these poor miserable people from the healthy, a measure which is considered wise, we have therefore ordered that a hospital should be built for them on a remote island. Provision has been made for the lepers' keep and it has been decided that all those who are admitted there should bring with them 20 daler, or goods to that value, for the benefit of the hospital. If neither they themselves nor their parents have sufficient means to pay the 20 daler, then the town or parish whence they came is obliged to find it. As this money accumulates it should be invested and the interest used to supplement the income of the hospital. We command that lepers already in hospital and those outside should be admitted to this hospital and remain there indefinitely, completely avoiding their family and friends and not mixing with any other healthy people. We also instruct our officials to have the country searched diligently, and if they have reason to believe that a person has been in close contact with someone who was infectious and who has since been admitted to hospital then, when it is verified, they must forbid him to mix with other people for at least one year, so that it can be ascertained whether he is free of the disease or not. The severest punishment and fines will be meted out to anyone who is caught breaking this law. Those infectious people who have been admitted to hospital will not be permitted to go into the towns or country in order to beg, because we have made appropriate provision for them. The clergy must be particularly instructed, on pain of strict punishment and fine, to ensure carefully both in town and country that as soon as someone is suspected to be infected the authorities are informed; he can then be isolated from others in good time and be admitted to hospital. The governor and sheriff are furthermore in duty bound to take charge of and to use with discretion the income provided for the support of the sick, so that none of the lepers in the hospital suffer hardship.

[1] Fagerlund (1886), pp. 23-25.

11. Reglemente för inrättningen—

Regulations of the leper hospital at Gloskär in the Åland islands, drawn up by Per Brahe, Regent of Finland, 1653[1]

As the hospital buildings on Åland are completed and the sick are already assembled there we have deemed it necessary to entrust the rural dean, the Reverend Boëtius Muur, and the sheriff on Åland, the honourable and worshipful Staphan Hansson, with the inspection of the hospital concerning the needs of those poor people, so that the godly work may be in good hands. They must pay attention to the following stipulations:—

1. The rules must be stricly obeyed year by year and the sick must be provided with the necessary firewood and food. A good warden must take up permanent residence in a separate house on the same island, either alone or at the most with one other to deputise in case of illness.
2. The food and firewood regulations must be written up in all three buildings and the fuel must be carefully eked out otherwise they could die of hunger and cold.
3. The warden is entitled to a small boat provided and maintained by the hospital, but he must not use it further afield than to the church and vicarage. He must not use it for skulduggery or for begging in the villages. When the boat is not required for official business it must be locked up so that the sick cannot under any circumstances make off.
4. The infectious[2] must bring with them cooking utensils, bedclothes, everyday clothes and their own keep, as far as their means verified at the parish meeting allow.
5. If they lack cloth, yarn, shoes or socks the warden must ask the priest to note down their deficiencies in detail. The sheriff's officer is to pass this list on to the sheriff, and when he has procured the necessary items they are to be distributed by the warden in the presence of a trustworthy man.
6. Almsboxes are to be placed in all harbours.... The money is to be collected twice a year, at midsummer and in the autumn. The priest should record the contents and the sheriff must hand on both the list and the money to the hospital.
7. A copy of the statement of the hospital's finances kept by the sheriff must be posted in several churches for information and questioning. At least every other year the dean and the sheriff must visit the hospital and inspect.
8. The sick are entitled to have their own scales with which to check on the warden's honesty.

[1] Fagerlund (1886), pp. 157-159.

[2] All those admitted were considered to be lepers: the document refers to the inmates indiscriminately as "the sick" or "the infectious".

9. The warden is not allowed to be away from the island on his own or hospital business for longer than twenty-four hours at a time.
10. The warden is forbidden on pain of severe punishment to mix even casually with the sick either on the island, in their dwellings, on outlying farms, or in the church pews; he must keep himself somewhat apart. He will be punished for carelessness and infidelity if he is apprehended and convicted.
11. The sick should boldly tell the parish priests when they visit both what they get and what they lack. The priests must pass the information on to the dean and to the sheriff.
12. It must be ensured that alms sent from the harbours and from charitable people are received by everyone who is entitled to them. The alms are to be put in boxes and the warden is to receive two or three times as much, according to what the inspectors deem fair.

Other matters, such as details of church services, funerals or anything else must be referred to the dean.... Any matters within the jurisdiction of the cathedral chapter should be referred there for decision. These regulations must be observed by all those who are concerned.

Per Brahe,
Stockholm, May 23rd, 1653.

12. Förslag till stat för Gammelstads hospital i Helsingfors.

Proposal for the budget of Gammelstads hospital, Helsingfors, 1651[1]

The regulations of the Mayor and Council in Helsingfors for the lepers in the hospital of this town, their upkeep and monthly allowance, drawn up on March 4th, 1651.

On the above date there are in this hospital, God help us, 20 persons, men and women, infected with the said dangerous and infectious disease. Each person ought to receive the following as one month's allowance....

Their family shall, as long as they live, provide the requisite clothes and shoes. If they have no family or their family is unable to help in this way, then they must be provided according to their need from the cashbox, provided the warden has previously obtained the administrator's permission to make this dispensation. As far as the monthly food and other provisions are concerned the administrator shall distribute them as follows:

1. Early each month he is to distribute these things to the poor, and if there is insufficient in kind he must obtain from the hospital's funds money according to the Crown's valuation with which to purchase the shortfall from elsewhere, so that the poor suffer no ill or want of food. The administrator must grind the rye to flour: two parts are to be used for baking bread and the third part is to be used as cooking flour. The third part of the barley must be made into malt—one barrel each month, from which four barrels of small beer are to be brewed, of which the poor are to receive one barrel each week. The remaining ten bushels of barley are to be made into grain which must be shared between them as far as it allows, according to the above regulations.
2. He must take trouble in every respect to keep the poor people's accounts carefully, and to enter everything correctly, both what he himself receives as gifts from good christian folk in God's name, as well as what he takes out on their behalf from the Crown's provisions and funds.
3. He must not forget to make a note of the day and date when somebody dies, and to keep a record of the part of their monthly food thus saved.
4. He must take great care that when a leper is brought to the hospital he be not admitted until he has given the warden, for the benefit of the poor, 20 daler in silver together with one month's provisions according to the royal ordinance; if he himself or his relatives are unable to raise the money, then the town or village whence he came must pay before he is admitted.
5. He must not be discouraged from travelling into the country once a year, particu-

[1] Sandholm (1973), pp. 433-435.

larly in autumn and winter, to solicit help from christian folk for the upkeep of the poor, according to the instructions he is to be given in due course.

6. He is obliged to render an annual account to the mayor and council in the presence of Philip Jacobsen, the honorable governor or his deputy, both of the monthly food allowance and also of gifts and other income in money or in goods, because the hospital finances must be put right once and for all, so that capital can accumulate as at other places, by means of which they can generously be supported.

7. And finally, when the administrator has carried out and completed his duty according to these instructions with all proven faithfulness and great diligence, he shall first expect thanks and secondly receive an annual salary. If on the contrary he is found to have been careless or unfaithful in any respect, he shall not only lose his wages but shall in addition be fined for such negligence according to the law, and shall suffer the magistrate's displeasure. The above instructions are to be followed both by him and by others whom it may concern.

13. Stat och Spijs ordning för Siählöö Hospital—

Budget for Sjählö leper hospital and mental hospital, Finland, by decree of King Carl XI of Sweden, May 6th, 1695[1]

				4	5	6
Per person for 1 year						
4 T:r[2]	12 cappar[3]	grain at $2\frac{1}{4}$ D:4[4]		9:	28:	$19\frac{1}{5}$:
4 Llb[7]	16m[8] meat			3:	19:	$4\frac{4}{5}$:
2 Llb	8m salt			1:	6:	$9\frac{3}{5}$:
2 Llb	12m butter			—:	31:	$4\frac{4}{5}$:
3 Llb	herring			—:	24:	—:
				16	13	$14\frac{2}{5}$:
For 3 festivals						
9 cappar	grain			—:	21:	$14\frac{2}{5}$:
6m	meat			—:	7:	$4\frac{4}{5}$:
3m	butter			—:	7:	$19\frac{1}{5}$:
$1\frac{1}{2}$m	hops			—:	3:	$14\frac{2}{5}$:
For fish				—:	3:	—:
				1	11	$4\frac{4}{5}$:
$1\frac{1}{2}$ armfulls of pinewood from the shore for cooking and firewood				—:	12:	—:
For shoes				—:	23:	8 :
			Total	18:	28:	$3\frac{1}{5}$:
			Total for 60 persons	1132:	24:	—:
For wine and sacramental wafers in hospital and church				12:	—:	—:
For Christmas candles at the same places $\frac{1}{2}$ Llb tallow					26:	—:
Contribution to the support of the poor in Åbo						
50 T:r grain at $2\frac{1}{4}$ Dal.				112:	16:	—:

[1] Fagerlund (1886), pp. 42–47. This statute remained in force until 1814.

[2] T:r = *Tunnor*; the size of a ton varied slightly between different countries and even between different cities in the same country. The Swedish ton referred to here was approximately equal to the English ton (2240 pounds). For further details see Gerhardt (1798).

[3] 32 *Cappar* = 1 ton.

[4] *Daler*.

[5] *Öre*.

[6] *Pennia*: 1 *daler* = 32 *öre* = 24 *pennia*.

[7] *Llb* = *Lispund* which was 20 pounds; the Swedish pound was larger (500 g) than the English pound (454 g).

[8] m = *Mark*; there were 3 different Swedish marks of weight, all a little less than 1 pound.

To the hospital's priest for subsistence and salary						
Money	132:	16:	—:			
30 T:r grain at $2\frac{1}{4}$ Dal.	67:	16:	—:	200:	—:	—:
To the warden at the same place						
Money	103:	24:	—:			
25 T:r grain at $2\frac{1}{4}$ Dal.	56:	8:	—:			
For paper and ink purchased	5:	—:	—:	165:	—:	—:
To the bell-ringer who is also a priest						
Money	39:	—:	—:			
16 T:r grain at $2\frac{1}{4}$ Dal.	36:	—:	—:	75:	—:	—:
To the boy who acts as messenger as salary				12:	—:	—:
The miller receives 4 T:r grain in return for which he is to grind all the hospital's grain without further charge				9:	—:	—:
The blacksmith receives 2 T:r grain				4:	16:	—:
To each 4 servants on the hospital's farm 4 T:r grain at $2\frac{1}{4}$ Dal.	9:	—:	—:			
half a slaughter cow for meat and shoeleather	2:	—:	—:			
2 Llb 8m salt	1:	6:	$9\frac{3}{5}$:			
12m butter	—:	31:	$4\frac{4}{5}$:			
4 Llb 16m herring	1:	6:	$9\frac{3}{5}$:			
Total	14:	12:	—:			
Total for 4 persons	57:	16:	—:			
Wages for each boy						
Money	5:	—:	—:			
Stedsell	1:	—:	—:			
For 2 shirts	1:	8:	—:			
3m wool for stockings and gloves	—:	16:	—:			
1 pair of work gloves	—:	8:	—:			
Total	8:	—:	—:			
Total for 2 boys	16:	—:	—:			
Wages for each girl						
Money	3:	10:	16:			
Stedsell	—:	16:	—:			
Linen	1:	8:	—:			
2m wool for stockings and gloves	—:	10:	16:			
Total	5:	13:	8:			
Total for 2 girls	10:	26:	16:	84:	10:	16:

To the foreman of the clean poor (who is one of them and obtains his keep with them) for looking after the mentally sick in the madhouse	6:	—:	—:
To the foreman of the unclean or lepers at the same place	4:	—:	—:
The watchman at Kupis well receives altogether 3 T : r corn at $2\frac{1}{4}$ Dal.	6:	24:	—:
For the poor people's coffins at $21\frac{1}{3}$ öre, repairs to the church and necessary incidental expenses on the farm as much as is required is granted if the accounts appear to be correctly paid			
Although this budget is formulated for 60 persons, the lord lieutenant and the bishops may admit as many more as the funds allow, but care must be taken to retain some of the income as capital which can be lent out on interest against a security.			
Grand Total	1824:	24:	16:

14. Extract from a letter written to Johannes Petersen in 1767 by Joen Givertsen, a priest suffering from leprosy in Iceland[1]

My disease is steadily progressing, which the chief physician of Iceland,[2] Biarne Poulsen, calls *Dispositionem Scorbutico Leprosam.* Three years ago I developed scabies[3] both on hands and feet, which continued until last winter when it disappeared, but in its place little lumps or nodules have appeared on my feet, upper leg, arms and face. My face is beginning to swell, however the colour is not yet very blue or dark, from which I conclude that my blood is not yet badly corrupted, which I attribute to the medicaments I have received from the well-known chief physician. Some time ago I started to drink *Decoctum* of *Trifolio Aquatico* and to eat *Cochleare*, after which I was no worse.

Three years ago a deep sore appeared on my left knee, which healed after a while but last year broke out again, whereupon I opened up the sore myself and have continually kept it clean from the fluid flowing from it. In the same knee and almost the whole of my thigh I have lost all sensation so that one could even put a hot or cold iron on it without me feeling it. The loss of sensation is just as great on the soles of my feet.

I cannot yet complain of difficulty in breathing although my voice has for some time become weaker; on the other hand what troubles me most at present is a very severe and almost insufferable pain in my feet, so that I can hardly bear to stay in bed. When they become warm they usually begin to swell, a swelling which rapidly waxes and wanes. My feet are also a very bad colour with dark spots.

In the second year I took baths and also made a foot-bath of juniper wood, but I cannot bear this any longer. I have also applied leeches to both my arms and legs, but in vain.

[1] Petersen, J. (1769), pp. 24–26.

[2] *Land-Physicus*, was a state appointment. Poulsen was an experienced doctor with a wide experience of leprosy from his journeys through Iceland. See "Vice-Lavmand Eggert Olaffens og Landphysic Biarne Povelsens Reise igiennem Island". Soroe, 1772.

[3] *Scabies crustosa*, a skin infestation with the itch-mite.

15. En Klagesang—A Lament[1]

by Peder Olsen Feidie, patient in St. George's hospital for lepers, Bergen, from 1832 to 1849[2]

One wish my God I humbly make:
Help and spare me for Jesus' sake—
Say yes O God to this.
Grant my ever earnest desire
And with your grace my thoughts inspire;
Mould my thoughts as I now write
And give them clear expression.

This is my urgent daily prayer:
Forsake me not O God, draw near
For I am weak and frail.
Great anguish is within my heart,
Increases and will not depart;
My head with pain is heavy,
My eyes are growing dim.

I dream of when I was a lad,
Of all the happy times I had—
A joy it was to live.
But fortune quickly changed her face
And sorrow then did joy replace.
For me and many more
This fate has lain in store.

I was not yet fifteen years old,
My mind was full of joys untold,
Then were they all cut short.
Pain overcame me and did start
Quickly to pierce marrow bone and heart.
Oh! it was hard to bear
This burden laid on me.

Then for my father God did send,
His misery now was at an end,
His days on earth were done.

[1] Quoted by H. P. Lie in an unpublished manuscript "Spedalskhetens Historie i Norge", p. 254 ff, in the University of Bergen Library.

[2] The dates of Feidie's admission and death were found in the original hospital admissions book by L. J. Irgens in 1973.

Four children stood around the grave
And watched with silent faces brave,
As his tired bones were laid
In their earthy resting place.

As 'tis written we now must say
As Abraham asked Lot "Which way?—
Which way will you now take?
Pray take the left hand or the right
but beg our herdsmen not to fight".
Oh, save us now we pray
From all such strife to-day.

From one another we must part
For it was clear in mother's heart
That I was burdensome.
Long hours of vigil has she kept,
And often times till weak has wept
O'er me and other trials,
As you know best, O Lord.

This heavy cross must fall on me
As tempest roars tumultuously
To sink ship and cargo.
Thus sailors cry in sore distress,
O help us Lord for we are lost,
In truth I hope to find
A haven 'gainst all storm.

For other illnesses found here
Wise doctors on the scene appear,
Who understand disease.
To hospital those sick are brought,
And for their plight a cure is sought.
Thus their ills are relieved,
And all their wounds are dressed.

We lepers can no doctors get:
Here must we stay and wait and fret,
Until our time is up.
Peter from prison did escape
Because on God's grace he did wait.
O God, break now the chains
Which bind our limbs with pains.

Sometimes I softly walk about
The silent house at evening time:
Sorrowful sounds I hear.
One bitterly cries "woe is me"
Another sighs and groans that he
must creep away to bed.
Tell me O God—how long?

One is covered with sore on sore,
Another is dumb—speaks no more,
A third hobbles on crutches.
A fourth no daylight now can see,
A fifth has lost all his fingers.
Surely now it is clear
What we must suffer here?

In St. George's Hospital here,
Sufferings over a hundred bear,
And wait to be set free.
O holy Ghost our Helmsman true,
Steer us all our sufferings through,
And to heaven lead us,
For there are we set free.

It is the blind's hope and belief,
Their cries burst out for this relief,
That God will give them sight.
So now I pray God for my eyes
To soothe the pain which in them lies,
The best salve of them all
Made from the fish's gall.

Now after Jesus we must call—
O Lord have mercy, save us all—
As the woman once cried.
This is our punishment for sin,
Therefore we cannot hope to win
More than a few small crumbs
Of mercy from Thy grace.

But even if our health be lost,
Yet are we not from God's sight tossed—
That can we daily see
Wonderful gifts to us God sends,
Provides us with kind, unknown friends—
Both rich and poor are they.
O Lord do them repay.

Let us now humbly thank all those
Who with their time and caring chose
To give us such a house.
It was my fate and many other's,
Banished from sisters and from brothers,
From our homes to be tossed
Because our health was lost.

Just so that everyone can see
That God cares for us tenderly,
Thus are we sorely scourged.
He give and takes just as he will,

So take Lord from us our poor souls;
When from here we wander
Bring us to heaven's shore.

The angel rippled waters cool,
The first man in Siloam's pool
Was cured of all his ills.
Thus are we cleansed in sorrow's tears,
Which from our weeping eyes do flow
For the day we shall flee
This place of misery.

May God to suffering comfort bring,
As surely as the joy of Spring
Follows winter darkness:
When we shall see that shining light
Which bathes God's mercy-stool so bright.
O joy without an end,
Comfort in misery send.

So I advise you one and all
This our example to recall—
Rely not on yourselves.
Be not as Pilate when he spake
With Jesus standing at his feet,
Strong in his earthly power
To judge him in that hour.

Nobody else doth it concern,
God only doth the tasks discern
Within his vineyard here.
On some he sets a golden crown,
On some he lays a heavy cross;
A plot each man receives
To till as best he can.

So fare you well my sorry state,
In heaven lies our true estate,
Thither we long to go.
Judas here doth men's hearts harden;
The world in truth is our garden.
Such are the twinéd ropes
Which fetter all men's hope.

So now I end my humble song,
O God let not the time be long—
Thy will be done O Lord.
My wish it is, I who am weak,
After my death Thy throne to seek,
To praise Thee and behold
Thy countless joys untold.

16. Law regarding the isolation of people infected with leprosy and their confinement in public hospital in Iceland, 1898[1]

We Christian the Ninth, by the grace of God king of Denmark, lord of the Vends and Goths, duke of Schlesvig, Holstein, Stormarn, Ditmarsken, Lauenburg and Oldenburg make known:

The *Althing* (Icelandic Parliament) has resolved and We with Our consent have established the following law:

1. District and assistant physicians have each in his district to keep a record of all lepers in accordance with the requirements of the chief officer of health, who in turn is to confer with the physician of the leper hospital. The expenses in connection with the purchase of the said books of reference are to be borne by the state treasury.

Once every year the physician must present to the chief officer of health an extract of the book of reference in accordance with his further instructions.

2. When people affected with leprosy remove from one district to another the physician in the first district is to announce such removal to the physician in the other district.

3. The physician must each in his district keep a close watch on the way of life of those affected with leprosy in their respective districts. They have to inform those affected and those living together with them of all the necessary directions about what is to be observed, both by those affected and those not affected in order to avoid contamination, and to see to it that all these directions are observed. The parish alderman and the sanitary commissioner have to assist the physician in all possible ways to that purpose.

4. The lepers must always comply with the following instructions:

(1) Lepers must not share a bed with others, married couples forming an exception unless the physician should give directions to the contrary.

(2) Every leper should have a spittoon of his own and he is not allowed to spit on the floor.

(3) He shall have special cooking utensils, eating utensils and table furniture of every description, which only he must use.

(4) Lepers' bedding and wardrobe, cooking utensils, eating utensils and table furniture should be cleaned and washed separately. Their wound dressings should be burned after use or disinfected by boiling in water for at least one half hour.

(5) Lepers are prohibited to nurse children, to wait upon non-lepers, and to cook for others.

[1] Lepra, 1900, 1, 152–154.

(6) Lepers are prohibited, unless it is essential, to visit other farmsteads or to receive visits from others. It is likewise his duty to observe further precautions which the physicians, according to circumstances, may consider necessary and practicable.

5. Room or rooms which a leper has occupied must not be occupied by others before disinfection directed by the physician. The same applies to wardrobe, bedding or the like which has been used by a leper.

6. When a leper dies or removes to another place it is the duty of the landlord immediately to announce the fact to the sheriff or police chief who, within the space of 14 days, must himself inform the physician. The latter must thereupon without delay take the necessary steps to have the leper's room or rooms, wardrobe and bedding, as well as other articles of use which he may have left behind, properly disinfected.

7. Lepers receiving assistance from the institution for the relief of the poor must, if the district physician finds it necessary, be removed to the hospital for lepers. Should such removal not take place the patients in question must be put in a place which offers the greatest probability that the directions contained in paragraph 4 are strictly followed. The arrangements made for such lepers must, if circumstances allow, be such that married couples are not separated against their will. Should the decision taken by the physician cause such separation, it is only valid when endorsed by the prefect.

Children of leprous parents who are receiving assistance from the institution for the relief of the poor should always be brought up in other homes. Without the consent of the physician the parish council must not place paupers in any home where lepers are living.

8. Upon the request of the parish council and physician it is within the power of the prefect, in exceptional cases, to order the removal of other lepers to the hospital for lepers. This can only take place when either the instructions and further precautions mentioned in paragraph 4 are not satisfactorily observed, or in the opinion of the physician the disease or the danger of infection is so serious that removal to the hospital is necessary. Also in the cases dealt with in this paragraph care is to be taken that married couples are not separated unless absolutely necessary.

9. If necessary, removal to the hospital according to the present law must be executed by the police.

10. All expenses in connection with the lepers sojourn in the hospital for lepers, as well as all expenses in connection with the removal of patients under paragraph 8, are to be borne by the state treasury. As to the removal to the hospital for lepers under paragraph 7 the costs are to be born by the municipal authorities. The expenses in connection with the repeated removal of a patient who has left the hospital without permission of the hospital authorities must be borne by himself, as far as he is in a position to pay.

11. For journeys which the physicians may undertake in compliance with this law they are entitled to payment as for journeys and business in public service. All outlays and expenses incurred by disinfection under paragraph 6 are borne by the state treasury.

12. Transgression of those instructions contained in paragraph 5 as well as failure to comply with the duty of reporting laid down in paragraph 6 is punishable with

fines of up to 200 kroner. All cases concerning such transgressions are treated in the public police court.

13. This law is to come into force three months after the day upon which public announcement has been made that the hospital for lepers is, or from a certain specified moment will be, ready for use, which announcement should appear in the government gazette part B.

This is to be observed by all those persons, whom it may concern.

Given at Amalienborg in Copenhagen 4. February, 1898.

Ministry for Iceland.

17. Letter from President Relander of Finland to the lepers in Orivesi hospital after his visit in January 1930

To you who suffer,

You have been given a heavy burden in life but try to face it the right way. Do not despair, do not become hard, do not lose faith in life. In everything there is a purpose, even in your suffering.

Try to understand this. Do not forget the true secret of a happy life. Lasting happiness is never to be found merely in outward things. True happiness is only attained by the one who has the peace of God in his heart.

Behind dark clouds the clear sun is shining; after night the dawn breaks. So it will be with you when you learn to understand it, when the meaning of your hard fate at last becomes clear to you. Then you will see your sorrow as a great blessing. Then you will have found the great love of God and His love will have found you.

CHAPTER NOTES

Works listed in the Select Bibliography are not quoted in full in these notes.

Introduction. Leprosy

1. This is a personal view of a very controversial issue: a useful summary of evidence of syphilis in Europe before Columbus is given by B. L. Gordon in *Medieval and Renaissance Medicine*, London 1960, pp. 524–538.

I. A Cross-roads in History

1. Boëtius Murenius, *Acta visitatoria 1637–1666*, Finska Kyrkohistoriska Samfundets Handlingar VI, Helsingfors 1917. For details of Muur himself see Väinö Perälä, *Boëtius Murenius, lektor vid Åbo gymnasium och kontraktsprost på Åland*, Mariehamn 1910.
2. Rachel Reader, "New Evidence for the Antiquity of Leprosy in Early Britain", *Journal of Archaeological Science*, 1974, **1**, 205–207.
3. W. Bonser, *The Medical Background of Anglo Saxon England*, London 1963.
4. J. Y. Simpson (1841), p. 311.
5. A. F. Grön (1953), p. 151.
6. For an excellent summary of leprosy in literature see S. N. Brody (1974), pp. 147–197. In the previous chapter he traces theological interpretations of the disease concluding (p. 146): "... the medieval poets inherited an ancient and persuasive tradition that branded the leper as a pariah. It accused him of being immoral, separated him from society, took him as a figure of sin, feared him for the disease he spread and for the terror he inspired. It is this background that shapes the literary representation of the leper as a man who is morally depraved, whose body bears the stain of his spiritual corruption."
7. G. Chaucer, *The Canterbury Tales*, translated into modern English by N. Coghill, p. 26. London 1960.
8. R. Henryson, *The Testament of Cresseid*, edited by D. Fox, London 1968. The quotations here from Fox's edition have been rendered into modern English by the author with the assistance of D. S. Brewer.
9. Second Report of the Committee on Devonshire Folklore, in *Transactions of the Devon Association*, 1877, **9**, 88–102.
10. R. M. Clay (1966), p. 251.
11. C. Creighton (1965), p. 107.
12. Document 3.
13. J. Cule (1970), p. 44.
14. L. W. Fagerlund (1886), p. 183.

II. The Lepers of Åland

1. L. W. Fagerlund (1886), p. 288.
2. L. W. Fagerlund (1886), p. 261.
3. L. W. Fagerlund (1886), p. 279.
4. L. W. Fagerlund (1886), p. 285.
5. Document 11.

III. Bread, Beer, and Firewood

1. See J. F. D. Shrewsbury, *A History of the Bubonic Plague in the British Isles*, Cambridge 1971.
2. J. E. Welhaven (1816), p. 215.
3. Documents 2–4.
4. The food regulations for Själö hospital in 1695, which remained in force until 1814, still gave special allowances at Christmas, Easter and Whitsun—see Document 13.

IV. Means of Support

1. The records are confusing because it is often not specified whether the payment was made in silver or copper coin. In 1619, the admission fee to Själö hospital was 20 silver or 60 copper daler. The fee was the same at Helsingfors in 1651, and as late as 1739 20 silver daler were collected for a leper in Viitasaari. In 1763, the hospital admission fee was increased to 100 silver daler (see Å. Sandholm (1973), p. 173). Muur quotes a fee of 50 daler (presumably in copper coin), a sum which may indicate that the fee was reduced on Åland in response to public outcry.
2. Document 13.
3. Document 1.
4. R. M. Clay (1966), p. 135.
5. Document 7.
6. R. M. Clay (1966), p. 189.
7. R. M. Clay (1966), p. 193.

V. Sentence and Certificates

1. G. de Chauliac, *Inventarium sive Collectium Artis Chirurgicalis Medicinae*, Avignon 1363.
2. Document 8.
3. J. Y. Simpson (1842), pp. 150–151.
4. L. W. Fagerlund (1886), pp. 255–256.
5. Å. Sandholm (1974), p. 51.
6. E. Windeatt (1880), p. 463.
7. Document 9.

VI. Separation

1. Document 1.
2. C. Creighton (1965), p. 102.
3. H. T. Riley, *Memorials of London and London Life*, London 1868, pp. 230–231.
4. Quoted by C. Platt, *The English Medieval Town*, London 1976, p. 70.
5. R. M. Clay (1966), p. 141.
6. Document 4.
7. Document 3.
8. P. V. Glob, *The Bog People*, London 1971, pp. 110–111.
9. P. Nørlund, *De Gamle Nordbobygder ved Verdens Ende*, 4th edition, Copenhagen 1967, pp. 99–121.
10. For a discussion of theories explaining the mysterious disappearance of the Norse Greenlanders in the fifteenth century see J. T. Oleson, *Early Voyages and Northern Approaches*, Toronto 1963, pp. 70–86; also H. Ingstad, *Land under the Polar Star*, London 1966, pp. 320–335.
11. J. Y. Simpson (1842), p. 420.
12. J. Y. Simpson (1842), p. 424.
13. E. L. Ehlers (1898), p. 25.

VII. Husbands and Wives

1. See S. N. Brody (1974), pp. 82–83.
2. J. Cule (1970), p. 40.
3. L. W. Fagerlund (1886), pp. 98–99.

VIII. Despair and Hope

1. Document 1.
2. The words used for "wood and nails for coffins" were *bräder och spiik til lijkkistor*—*lijk* is the same word as the English "lich" or "lych" meaning corpse, as in lych-gate, the place where a coffin awaited the arrival of the priest. On another occasion the word *dödkista* was used, and there is no doubt that the lepers were required to bring materials for the coffin in which they would be buried.
3. J. Y. Simpson (1842), p. 419.
4. L. W. Fagerlund (1886), p. 98.
5. See S. N. Brody (1974), pp. 107–146.
6. Document 15.
7. Document 3.
8. J. E. Welhaven (1816), p. 217.
9. J. Y. Simpson (1842), pp. 149–150.
10. J. L. Odhelius (1774), p. 267.
11. J. Y. Simpson (1842), p. 143.
12. L. W. Fagerlund (1886), pp. 48–49.
13. J. E. Welhaven (1816), p. 210.
14. J. E. Welhaven (1816), p. 214.
15. Document 15.
16. L. W. Fagerlund (1886), p. 152.
17. J. E. Welhaven (1816), p. 197.
18. Quoted by D. Fox in R. Henryson, *The Testament of Cresseid*, London 1968, p. 41.

IX. The Rise and Fall of the Disease

1. L. W. Fagerlund (1886), pp. 113–118.
2. E. Kaurin, "Leprastudier" in *Festskrift i anledning av overlæge dr. med. D.C. Danielssens 50 aarige Embedsjubileum*, Bergen 1891, p. 8.
3. P. S. Abraham, "Leprosy: a review of some facts and figures", in *Illustrated Medical News*, London May 25th 1889, p. 7.
4. J. Halenius, "Spetälskan eller Elfkarlebysjukan, såsom gängse i Elfkarleby socken, belängen vid Dalelfvens utmynning i Bottniska viken", *Collegii Medicii Berättelse*, Stockholm 1761. J. Hjorts, "Elephantiasis eller Elfkarlebysjukan såsom i mer och mindre grad nog allmän hos allmogen särdeles på östra och norra siden av landet", *Collegii Medicii Berättelse*, Stockholm 1796.
5. S. Talvik, *Die Lepra im Kreise Oesel*, Tartu 1921.
6. A. Spindler, "The pathogenesis of leprosy", *International Journal of Leprosy*, 1935, 3, 265–278.
7. Document 17.
8. G. Benediktsson and O. Bjarnason, *Nordisk Medicin*, 1959, **62**, 1225–1227.
9. L. J. Derbes, *Account of the Faroe Islands*, 1676, quoted by R. Liveing, *Elephantiasis graecorum or True Leprosy*, London 1873, pp. 29–30.
10. Document 16.
11. E. L. Ehlers (1895), p. 180.
12. E. L. Ehlers (1895), p. 184.
13. J. Y. Simpson (1842), pp. 142–143.
14. C. Engelbreth, *Spedalskhedens Oprindelse*, Copenhagen 1912, pp. 40–41.
15. T. R. B. Bucholz, *Spedalskheden som Folkesygdom*, Christiana 1872.

16. R. Liveing, *Elephantiasis or True Leprosy*, London 1873.
17. E. L. Ehlers (1895), pp. 169–170.
18. W. L. Washburn, "Leprosy among Scandinavian Settlers in the upper Mississipi valley 1864–1932", *Bulletin of the History of Medicine*, 1950, **24**, 123–148.
19. G. H. A. Hansen, "On the prevention of emigration and immigration of lepers", *Lepra*, 1900, **1**, 88–89.

X. Leprosy—Fact or Fiction?

An unbroken chain

1. L. J. Derbes, *Account of the Faroe Islands*, 1676, quoted by R. Liveing, *Elephantiasis graecorum or True Leprosy*, London 1873, pp. 29–30.
2. H. Spöring (1738), p. 14.
3. W. H. Jopling, "Leprosy", *British Journal of Hospital Medicine*, 1974, **11**, 43–50.
4. I. Uddman (1765), p. 13.
5. Holland (1812), p. 202.
6. Document 14.
7. Hansen's discovery of clumps of bacilli in a leprous nodule was published in 1874 (G. H. A. Hansen, "Undersøgelser angående Spedalskhedens Årsager", *Norsk Magasin Lægevidenskap*, 1874, **3**, 76–78). Leprosy bacteria were only the second bacteria causing human disease to be described. The first, anthrax, were identified in 1870 by the German pathologist Robert Koch, who in 1882 caused another sensation with his discovery of the cause of tuberculosis.

Pictorial evidence

8. A. R. Hall, *The Scientific Revolution 1500–1800*, London 1954, p. 45.
9. J. Y. Simpson (1842), p. 144.
10. H. P. Lie (undated), *Spedalskhetens Historie i Norge*, (unpublished).
11. One volume recorded topography, another, the *Zoological and Medical Atlas*, included the lepers as the only medical plates. See P. Gaimard (1838–52).

Graveyard proof

12. See V. Møller-Christensen (1951) and (1953).
13. See V. Møller-Christensen (1961) and J. G. Andersen (1969).
14. The anterior nasal spine is a small spur of bone which lies under the cartilage which devides the nostrils.
15. R. Melsom, "Changes in the maxillary bone in leprosy", *International Journal of Leprosy*, 1953, **21**, 617.
16. M. F. Lechat, "Bone lesions in leprosy", *International Journal of Leprosy*, 1962, **30**, 125–137.
17. J. G. Andersen (1969), pp. 92–95.
18. See V. Møller-Christensen (1958).
19. V. Møller-Christensen, "Case of leprosy from the Middle Ages of Denmark", *Acta Medica Scandinavica*, 1952, **142**, Supplement 266, 101–108.
20. C. Creighton (1965), pp. 237–279.
21. K. Isager, *Skeletfundene ved Øm kloster*, København, 1936.
22. V. Møller-Christensen (1958), p. 136.
23. C. Creighton (1965), pp. 72–76.
24. V. Møller-Christensen (1963), pp. 41–47.

SELECT BIBLIOGRAPHY

Andersen, J. G. (1969). *Studies in the mediaeval diagnosis of leprosy in Denmark*. M.D. Thesis, Copenhagen.

Birch, W. de G. (1887). *Catalogue of seals in the Department of manuscripts in the British Museum*, vol. 1. London.

Bonser, W. (1963). *The medical background of Anglo-Saxon England*. London.

Bracken, H. M. (1900). "Leprosy in Minnesota". *Lepra*, **1**, 37–43.

Brody, S. N. (1974). *The Disease of the Soul: leprosy in medieval literature*. Cornell University Press: Ithaca.

Browne, S. G. (1970). "Leprosy". *Documenta Geigy Acta Clinica* No. 11.

Clay, R. M. (1909). *The Mediaeval Hospitals of England*, reprinted 1966. Cass: London.

Creighton, C. (1965). "Leprosy in medieval Britain". Chapter II in *A History of Epidemics in Britain*, second edition, vol. 1, pp. 69–113. Cass: London.

Cule, J. (1970). "The diagnosis, care and treatment of leprosy in Wales and the border in the Middle Ages". *Transactions of the British Society for the History of Pharmacy*, **1**, 29–58.

Ehlers, E. L. (1895). "On the conditions under which leprosy has declined in Iceland and the extent of its former & present prevalence". In *Leprosy Prize Essays*, pp. 153–187. The New Sydenham Society: London.

Ehlers, E. L. (1898). "Danske St. Jørgensgaarde i Middelalderen". *Bibliotek før Læger*, **1**, 243–288, 331–371, 639–644. Quoted here from reprint of 1898.

Fagerlund, L. W. (1886). *Finlands Leprosorier I*. Akademisk Afhandling: Helsingfors.

Fagerlund, L. W. (1903). "Finlands Leprosorier II. I. Maria Magdalenae, Wiborgs Hospital". In *Finska Vetenskaps-Societetens Bidrag*, **62**, 101–155.

Gaimard, P. (1838–52). *Voyage en Islande et au Groënland; Zoological and Medical Atlas*. Paris.

Gerhardt, M. R. B. (1798). "Almindelig Contorist eller den nyeste og for nærværende tid brygelige Mynt, Maal of Vægt Forfatning". *I. Europa*. Kobenhavn.

Grön, F. (1953). "Remarks on the earliest medical conditions in Norway and Iceland with special reference to British influence". In *Science, Medicine and History*, edited by E. A. Underwood, pp. 143–153. Oxford University Press: London.

Hansen, G. H. A. (1900). "On the prevention of emigration and immigration of lepers". *Lepra*, **1**, 88–99.

Hansen, G. H. A. and Lie, H. P. (1909). "Die Geschichte der Lepra in Norwegen". *II Internationale Wissenschaftliche Lepra-Konferenz Mitteilungen und Verhandlungen*, **1**, 52–78.

Holland (initial not given) (1812). "On the diseases of Iceland. Medical extracts no. VIII: From Sir G. S. Mackenzie's Travels". *Edinburgh Medical and Surgical Journal*, **8**, 201–207.

Hutchinson, W. (1787). *History of Durham*, vol. 1. Victoria County Histories.

Isager, K. (1936). *Skeletfundene ved Om Kloster*. Kobenhavn.

Martin, A. R. (1760). "Anmärkningar öfver den så kallade Spitelska Fisk och Boskap i Norrige". *Kungliga Svenska Vetenskaps Academiska Handlingar*, **21**, 306–311.

Møller, H. (1784). "Forsøg i det som angaaer det Norske Folks Sundhed". *Konglige Norske Videnskaps Selskapets Handlinger*, **1**, 193–262.

Møller-Christensen, V. (1951). "Om udgravningen af Næstved Sct. Jørgensgård i Aaderup". *Medicinsk Forum*, **4**, 1–16.

Møller-Christensen, V. (1952). "Case of leprosy from the Middle Ages of Denmark". *Acta Medica Scandinavica*, **142**, Supplement 266, 101–108.

Møller-Christensen, V. (1953). *Ten lepers from Næstved in Denmark*. Danish Science Press: Copenhagen.

Møller-Christensen, V. (1958). *Bogen om Æbelholt Kloster*. Dansk Videnskabs Forlag: København.

Møller-Christensen, V. (1961). *Bone changes in leprosy*. Munksgaard: Copenhagen.

Møller-Christensen, V. (1963). "Skeletfundene fra St. Jørgens Kirke i Svendborg". *Fynske Minder*, **5**, 35–49.

Newman, G. (1895). "On the history and the decline and final extinction of leprosy as an endemic disease in the British Islands". In *Leprosy Prize Essays*, pp. 1–150. The New Sydenham Society: London.

Odhelius, J. L. (1774). *Rön, om Lepra*. *Kungliga Svenska Vetenskaps Academiska Handlingar*, **35**, 266–271.

Paris, M. (1684). *Monachi Albanensis Angli, Historia Major*, edited by W. Watts. London.

Perälä, V. (1910). *Aland: Bidrag till Kännedom af hembygden utgifna af Föreningen Ålands Vanner, I*. Boëtius Murenius, lektor ved Abo gymnasium och kontrakspræst pa Åland, Mariehamn.

Petersen, J. (1769). *Den saakallede islandske Skiørbug*, Soroe.

Richards, P. (1960). "Leprosy in Scandinavia". *Centaurus*, 7, 101–133.

Robert, E. (1851). "Zoologie et Médecine". Unnumbered volume in series *Voyage en Islande et au Groënland, 1835–1836*, edited by P. Gaimard. Paris.

Sandholm, Å. (1973). "Kyrkan och Hospitalshjonen". *Finska Kyrko-historiska Samfundets Handlingar 88*. Helsingfors.

Sederholm, E. (1909). "History of Leprosy in Sweden". *II. Internationale Wissenschaftliche Lepra-Konferenz Mitteilungen und Verhandlungen*, **1**, 79–104.

Shapter, T. (1835). *A few observations on the Leprosy of the Middle Ages*. Exeter.

Simpson, J. Y. (1841). "Antiquarian notices of leprosy and leper hospitals in Scotland and England, part 1". *Edinburgh Medical and Surgical Journal*, 56, 301–330.

Simpson, J. Y. (1842). "Antiquarian notices of leprosy and leper hospitals in Scotland and England, parts 2 & 3". *Edinburgh Medical and Surgical Journal*, **57**, 121–156 and 394–429.

Spöring, H. D. (1738). "Observatio de Elephantiasi Aqua Martiali fontis Kupis, prope Aboam, curata, 1729". *Acta Literaria et Scientarium Sveciae*, 3, 14–16.

Strøm, H. (1784). "Anmmaerkninger til Oplysning om den ved Søekysterne i Norge gaengse Spedalskhed". *Konglige Norske Videnskaps Selskapets Handlinger*, **1**, 171–184.

Uddman, I. (1765). "Lepra, quam dissertatione medica, venia exper. facult. med. ad reg. acad. Upsal. praeside viro generosissimo Carolo von Linne. Upsaliae". Published in Swedish translation by E. Haglund in *Valda Avhandlingar av Carl von Linné*, Svenska Linné-Sällskapet Nr. 26, 1957.

Welhaven, J. E. (1816). "Beskrifning öfver de spetälske i St. Jörgens Hospital i staden Bergen i Norrige". *Svenska Läkare-Sällskapets Handlingar*, 3, 188–220.

Windeatt, E. (1880). "Some Religious Houses of Totnes". *Transactions of the Devon Association*, **12**, 455–463.

Index